CAMBRIDGE LIBRARY

Books of enduring scholarly value

Life Sciences

Until the nineteenth century, the various subjects now known as the life sciences were regarded either as arcane studies which had little impact on ordinary daily life, or as a genteel hobby for the leisured classes. The increasing academic rigour and systematisation brought to the study of botany, zoology and other disciplines, and their adoption in university curricula, are reflected in the books reissued in this series.

Arabian Medicine

E.G. Browne (1862–1926), who combined outstanding skills in medicine and Arabic and Persian studies, has left an indelible mark in his fields of expertise. He first learned Turkish in his teens, and went on to study all the languages of the Islamic tradition, while also qualifying as a physician. This collection of four FitzPatrick Lectures, delivered at the Royal College of Physicians in 1919–20, and first published in 1921, covers subjects such as Arabic as a scientific language, the transmission of Greek learning, and important Islamic medieval writers. Brown describes the role of Islamic physicians in transmitting Greek and Roman medical science through the Dark Ages, both preserving and building upon texts which were lost or misunderstood in the West. He further argues that the scientific elements of Islamic literature should be seen as complementing and supporting the imaginative and aesthetic works of literature, history and poetry.

Cambridge University Press has long been a pioneer in the reissuing of out-of-print titles from its own backlist, producing digital reprints of books that are still sought after by scholars and students but could not be reprinted economically using traditional technology. The Cambridge Library Collection extends this activity to a wider range of books which are still of importance to researchers and professionals, either for the source material they contain, or as landmarks in the history of their academic discipline.

Drawing from the world-renowned collections in the Cambridge University Library and other partner libraries, and guided by the advice of experts in each subject area, Cambridge University Press is using state-of-the-art scanning machines in its own Printing House to capture the content of each book selected for inclusion. The files are processed to give a consistently clear, crisp image, and the books finished to the high quality standard for which the Press is recognised around the world. The latest print-on-demand technology ensures that the books will remain available indefinitely, and that orders for single or multiple copies can quickly be supplied.

The Cambridge Library Collection brings back to life books of enduring scholarly value (including out-of-copyright works originally issued by other publishers) across a wide range of disciplines in the humanities and social sciences and in science and technology.

Arabian Medicine

*The FitzPatrick Lectures Delivered
at the College of Physicians in
November 1919 and November 1920*

E.G. BROWNE

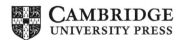
CAMBRIDGE
UNIVERSITY PRESS

CAMBRIDGE UNIVERSITY PRESS

Cambridge, New York, Melbourne, Madrid, Cape Town,
Singapore, São Paolo, Delhi, Mexico City

Published in the United States of America by Cambridge University Press, New York

www.cambridge.org
Information on this title: www.cambridge.org/9781108013970

© in this compilation Cambridge University Press 2012

This edition first published 1921
This digitally printed version 2012

ISBN 978-1-108-01397-0 Paperback

ARABIAN MEDICINE

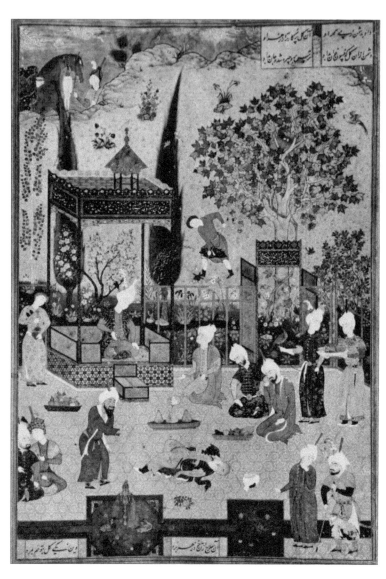

The Rival Physicians

(See pp. 89–90 of the text)

ARABIAN MEDICINE

BY

E. G. BROWNE

The FitzPatrick Lectures
delivered at the College of Physicians in
November 1919 and November 1920

CAMBRIDGE
AT THE UNIVERSITY PRESS
1962

PUBLISHED BY

THE SYNDICS OF THE CAMBRIDGE UNIVERSITY PRESS

Bentley House, 200 Euston Road, London, N.W. 1
American Branch: 32 East 57th Street, New York 22, N.Y.
West African Office: P.O. Box 33, Ibadan, Nigeria

First printed 1921
Reprinted 1962

First printed in Great Britain at the University Press, Cambridge
Reprinted by Bradford & Dickens, Ltd., London, W.C. 1

TO

SIR NORMAN MOORE, Bart., M.D.

PRESIDENT OF THE ROYAL COLLEGE OF PHYSICIANS

In admiration of his catholic scholarship, in gratitude for his inspiring teaching, and in memory of three fruitful years passed under his guidance at St Bartholomew's Hospital, I dedicate this book

PREFACE

In the course of the last ten years there have been conferred upon me two public honours which have given
me the greatest pleasure and satisfaction, my election
in 1911 as a Fellow of the Royal College of Physicians,
and the presentation, on the occasion of my fifty-ninth
birthday in February, 1921, of a complimentary address
(accompanied by very beautiful presents) signed by a
number of representative Persians, expressing their ap-
preciation of the services which, they were kind enough
to say, I had rendered to their language and literature.

I hope that this little book may be regarded, not as
a discharge, but as an acknowledgment, of this double
debt. In it I have sought on the one hand to indicate
the part played by the scholars and physicians of Islám,
and especially of Persia, in the transmission of medical
science through the dark ages from the decline of the
ancient to the rise of the modern learning; and on the
other to suggest to lovers of Arabic and Persian literature in the wider sense that hitherto they have perhaps
allowed the poets and euphuists to occupy a dispropor-
tionate amount of their attention, to the exclusion of
the scientific *Weltanschauung* which, to a greater degree
in the medieval East than in the modern West, forms
the background of these lighter, though more artistic,
efforts. Indeed, as I have attempted to show in these

pages[1], that great Persian poem the *Mathnawí* of
Jalálu'd-Dín Rúmí will be better appreciated by one
who is conversant with the medical literature of the
period.

Before I began to prepare the FitzPatrick lectures
now offered to the public I consulted Sir Clifford Allbutt,
the Regius Professor of Medicine in the University of
Cambridge, as to the best books on the history of that
science which the Prophet Muhammad, in a tradition
familiar to all Muslims, is said to have linked in importance with Theology[2]. Of the numerous works which
Sir Clifford Allbutt indicated, and, in many cases, lent
to me for preliminary study, I have derived more profit
from none than from Professor Max Neuburger's excellent *Geschichte der Medizin* (Stuttgart, 1908). Although
the section of this work dealing with Arabian Medicine
comprises only 86 pages[3], it is extraordinarily rich in
facts and accurate in details, and supplies an outline of
the subject which is susceptible of amplification but not
of correction.

I have thought it better to publish these four lectures
in the form in which they were originally delivered than
to recast them in a fresh mould, but the proofs have been
read by several of my friends and colleagues, namely
Dr F. H. H. Guillemard, M.D., Dr E. H. Minns, Litt.D.,

---

[1] See pp. 87–88 *infra*.

[2] "Science is twofold : Theology and Medicine."

اَلْعِلْمُ عِلْمَانِ عِلْمُ ٱلْأَدْيَانِ وَ عِلْمُ ٱلْأَبْدَانِ ‘

[3] Vol. I, part ii, pp. 142–228 = pp. 346–394 of vol. i of Ernest
Playfair's English translation (London, 1910).

Mírzá Muḥammad Khán of Qazwín, and Muḥammad Iqbál, to all of whom I am indebted for many valuable corrections and suggestions. I am also deeply indebted to Professor A. A. Bevan and the Rev. Professor D. S. Margoliouth for their help in establishing the text and emending the translation of the clinical case recorded by ar-Rází which will be found on pp. 51–3 *infra*.

It has afforded me particular pleasure to be allowed to dedicate this little volume explicitly to Sir Norman Moore, as representing that fine tradition of learning, acumen and humanity proper in all countries and ages to the great and noble profession of Medicine, with which living tradition, to my infinite advantage, I was brought in contact in my student days both here at Cambridge and in St Bartholomew's Hospital; and implicitly to those other great teachers in these two famous schools of medical learning whose methods of investigation and exposition I have endeavoured to apply in other fields of knowledge.

EDWARD G. BROWNE.

April 16, 1921.

CONTENTS

LECTURE I

THE extent of my subject and the limitations of the time at my disposal forbid me, even were it otherwise desirable, to introduce into these lectures any unessential or irrelevant matter. Yet I cannot lose this, the first opportunity accorded to me since my election as a Fellow of this College, of expressing publicly my deep sense of gratitude for an honour as highly appreciated as unexpected. I am well aware that this honour was conferred on me on the ground (the only ground on which it could have been conferred in my case) that, having regard to the position occupied by Arabian Medicine in the history of our profession, it was desirable that there should be amongst the Fellows of the College one who could study that system at first hand. There is a proverbial saying amongst the Arabs when the time comes when the services of a person or thing provided for a particular contingency are at last actually required—

ما أَدَّخَرْتُك يا دَمْعَتِى إلَّا لِشِدَّتِى—"*I have not stored thee up, O my tear, save for my time of distress*"; and when I was invited to deliver the FitzPatrick lectures this year, I felt that this proverb was applicable, and that, even though I felt myself unworthy of this fresh honour on the part of the College, it was impossible to decline, especially in view of the expressed wish of the President of the College, Sir Norman Moore, to whose inspiring teaching in my far-off student days I owe a greater debt of gratitude than I can adequately express. I can only hope that at the conclusion of my lectures you may not apply to me another proverbial saying of the Arabs:

مِنْ—أَوَّلِ غَزَوَاتِهِ ٱنْكَسَرَتْ عَصَاتُهُ—"*At the first bout his quarter-staff was broken.*"

When we speak of "Arabian Science" or "Arabian Medicine" we mean that body of scientific or medical doctrine which is enshrined in books written in the Arabic language, but which is for the most part Greek in its origin, though with Indian, Persian and Syrian accretions, and only in a very small degree the product of the Arabian mind. Its importance, as has long been recognized, lies not in its originality, but in the fact that in the long interval which separated the decay of Greek learning from the Renascence it represented the most faithful tradition of ancient Wisdom, and was during the Dark Ages the principal source from which Europe derived such philosophical and scientific ideas as she possessed. The translation of the Greek books into Arabic, either directly or through intermediate Syriac versions, was effected for the most part under the enlightened patronage of the early 'Abbásid Caliphs at Baghdád between the middle of the eighth and ninth centuries of our era by skilful and painstaking scholars who were for the most part neither Arabs nor even Muhammadans, but Syrians, Hebrews or Persians of the Christian, Jewish or Magian faith. Some four or five centuries later European seekers after knowledge, cut off from the original Greek sources, betook themselves with ever increasing enthusiasm to this Arabian presentation of the ancient learning, and rehabilitated it in a Latin dress; and for the first century after the discovery of the art of printing the Latin renderings of Arabic philosophical, scientific and medical works constituted a considerable proportion of the output of the European Press; until the revival of a direct knowledge of the

Greek originals in the first place, and the inauguration of a fresh, fruitful and first-hand investigation of natural phenomena in the second, robbed them to a great extent of their prestige and their utility, and changed the excessive veneration in which they had hitherto been held into an equally exaggerated contempt.

In recent years, however, when the interest and importance of what may be called the Embryology of Science has obtained recognition, the Arabian, together with other ancient and obsolete systems of Medicine, has attracted increasing attention, has formed the subject of much admirable and ingenious research, and has already produced a fairly copious literature. The chief Arabic biographical and bibliographical sources, such as the *Fihrist* or "Index" (377/987), al-Qifṭí's *History of the Philosophers* (c. 624/1227), Ibn Abí Uṣaybiʻa's *Classes of Physicians* (640/1242), the great bibliography of Ḥájji Khalífa (+1068/1658) and the like, have been made available in excellent editions, while their most essential contents have been summarized by Wenrich, Wüstenfeld, Leclerc, Brockelmann and others; the general character and relations of Arabian Medicine have been concisely yet adequately described by Neuburger, Pagel, Withington and Garrison, to name only a few of the more recent writers on the history of Medicine; while amongst more specialized investigations, to mention one branch only of the subject, the admirable works of Dr P. de Koning and Dr Max Simon have accurately determined the anatomical terminology of the Arabs and its equivalence with that of the Greek anatomists. For the pathological terminology much more remains to be done, and I have been greatly hampered in my reading of Arabic medical books by the difficulty of determining the exact scientific signification of many words used in

the ordinary literary language in a looser and less pre-
cise sense than that which they evidently bear in the
technical works in question. Nor is much help to be
derived from the medieval translations of the " Latino-
Barbari," who too often simply preserve in a distorted
form the Arabic term which they pretend to translate.
Thus the first section of the first discourse of the first
part of the third book of Avicenna's great *Qánún* is
entitled in the Latin Version *Sermo universalis de Sodâ*,
but who, not having the original before him, could
divine that *soda* stands for the Arabic صُداع, the ordinary
Arabic word for a headache, being the regularly formed
"noun of pain" from the verb صدع "to split"?

Now the history of Arabian Medicine can only be
studied in connection with the general history of Islám,
which, as you all know, first began to assume political
significance in A.D. 622. In that year Muḥammad,
whose real miracle was that he inspired the warring
tribes of Arabia with a common religious and social
ideal, welded them into one people, sent them forth
to conquer half the then known world, and founded an
Empire destined to rival and replace those of Caesar
and Chosroes, transferred the scene of his activities
from Mecca to al-Madína. This event marks the
beginning of the Muhammadan era known as the *hijra*
or "Flight," from which 1338 lunar years have now
elapsed. About the middle of this period, viz. in the
seventh century of the Flight and the thirteenth of our
era, Arabian or, more correctly speaking, Muhammadan Civilization suffered through the Mongol or
Tartar invasion an injury from which it never recovered,
and which destroyed for ever the Caliphate, the nominal
unity of the Arabian Empire, and the pre-eminence of

Baghdád as a centre of learning. Even before this, however, partly in consequence of the triumph of the narrower and more orthodox doctrines of the Ash'arí over the more liberal Mu'tazila school of theology, partly in consequence of the gradual displacement of Arabian and Persian by Turkish influences in the political world, science, and particularly philosophy (which was so closely connected with medicine that the title *Hakím* was, and still is, indifferently applied alike to the metaphysician and the physician), had ceased to be cultivated with the same enthusiasm and assiduity which had prevailed in "the Golden Prime of good Hárúnu'r-Rashíd" and his immediate predecessors and successors. This Golden Age of Arabian learning culminated in the century between A.D. 750 and 850, the century succeeding the establishment of the 'Abbásid Caliphate with its metropolis at Baghdád. Of the ten Caliphs who reigned during this period the second, al-Mansúr, and the seventh, al-Ma'mún (whose mother and wife were both Persians, and in whose reign Persian influences, already powerful, reached their culminating point), were conspicuous for their intellectual curiosity and for their love and generous patronage of learning, and for a broad tolerance which scandalized the orthodox and led one of them to change the Caliph's title of "Commander of the Faithful" (*Amíru'l-Mú'minín*) into that of "Commander of the Unbelievers" (*Amíru'l-Káfirín*)[1]. To the ancient learning, especially that of the ancient Greeks, they were enthusiastically attached; by purchase, conquest or exchange they possessed themselves of countless precious manuscripts, Greek and other, which they stored in the Royal Library or *Baytu'l-Hikmat* ("House of Wisdom") and caused to be

---

[1] 'Al-Ya'qúbí, ed. Houtsma, p. 546.

translated, by the most competent scholars they could attract to their court, into Arabic, either directly from the Greek, or through the intermédiary of the Syriac language. In the *Fihrist* or Index (*i.e.* of Sciences), an Arabic work composed in A.D. 987, more than a century after what I have spoken of as the "Golden Age," we have at once a mirror of the learning of that time, and an indicator of the appalling losses which it afterwards sustained, for of the books there enumerated it would hardly be an exaggeration to say that not one in a thousand now exists even in the most fragmentary form. The hateful Mongols—"that detestable nation of Satan," as old Matthew Paris (writing in A.D. 1240) calls them, "who poured forth like devils from Tartarus so that they are rightly called 'Tartars'"—did their work of devastation only too thoroughly, and the Muhammadan culture which survived the sack of Baghdád and the extinction of the Caliphate in A.D. 1258 was but a shadow of that which preceded it.

I have used the term "Muhammadan Civilization," which, for reasons to be given shortly, I prefer to "Arabian." As Latin was the learned language of medieval Europe, so was (and to some extent is) Arabic the learned language of the whole Muhammadan world. There is no objection to our talking of "Arabian Science" or "Arabian Medicine" so long as we never lose sight of the fact that this simply means the body of scientific or medical doctrine set forth in the Arabic language, for it is not until the eleventh century of our era that we begin to meet with what may be called a vernacular scientific literature in Muhammadan lands, a literature typified by such works as al-Bírúní's *Tafhím* on astronomy (eleventh century) and the *Dhakhíra* or

"Thesaurus" of Medicine composed for the King of Khwárazm or Khiva in the twelfth century.

Now this scientific literature in the Arabic language was for the most part produced by Persians, Syrians, Jews, and in a lesser degree by Greeks, but only to a very small extent by genuine Arabs. Ibn Khaldún, who composed his celebrated *Prolegomena to the Study of History*—one of the most remarkable books in Arabic—about A.D. 1400, judges his countrymen very harshly. He declares that every country conquered by them is soon ruined[1], that they are incapable of evolving a stable and orderly system of government[2], that of all people in the world they are the least capable of ruling a kingdom[3], and that of all people in the world they have the least aptitude for the arts[4]. Goldziher, one of the profoundest Arabic scholars of our time and himself a Jew, rightly says that Lagarde goes too far when he asserts that "of the Muhammadans who have achieved anything in science not one was a Semite"; yet he himself is constrained to admit that even in the religious sciences (exegesis of the *Qur'án*, tradition, jurisprudence, and the like) "the Arabian element lagged far behind the non-Arabian[5]." Much more evidence of this might be adduced, but I will content myself with one instance (hitherto, I believe, unnoticed in Europe) of the mistrust with which Arab practitioners of medicine were regarded even by their own people. The anecdote in question is related by that most learned but discursive writer al-Jáḥiẓ (so called on account of his prominent eyes) in his "Book of Misers" (*Kitábu'l-Bukhalá*[6]) and concerns an Arabian physician named

---

[1] De Slane's transl., i, p. 310. [2] *Ibid.*, i, p. 311.
[3] *Ibid.*, ii, p. 314. [4] *Ibid.*, ii, p. 365.
[5] See my *Lit. Hist. of Persia*, i, p. 260.
[6] Ed. Van Vloten, pp. 109–110.

Asad ibn Jání, who, even in a year of pestilence, and in spite of his recognized learning, skill and diligence, had but few patients. Being asked the reason of this by one of his acquaintances he replied: "In the first place I am a Muslim, and before I studied medicine, nay, before ever I was created, the people held the view that Muslims are not successful physicians. Further my name is Asad, and it should have been Salíbá, Mará'íl, Yuhanná or Bírá [*i.e.* a Syriac or Aramaic name]; and my *kunya* is Abu'l-Hárith, and it should have been Abú 'Ísá, Abú Zakariyyá or Abú Ibráhím [*i.e.* Christian or Jewish instead of Muhammadan]; and I wear a cloak of white cotton, and it should have been of black silk; and my speech is Arabic, and it should have been the speech of the people of Jundí-Shápúr" [in S.W. Persia].

The Arabs, whose scepticism was not confined to matters of religion, avenged themselves to some extent by disparaging verses about doctors, such as the following on the death of Yuhanná ibn Másawayhi (the Mesues of the medieval writers) in A.D. 857:

إنّ الطَّبِيبَ بِطِبّه و دوائه ، لا يستطيـع دفاعَ أَمْرٍ قد أَتى ،

ما للطبيب يموت بالدآء الّذى ، قد كان يُبْرِئُ منه فيما قد مضى ،

مات المداوِى و المداوَى و الّذى ، جلب الدوآء و باعه و مَن اشترى ،

"Verily the physician, with his physic and his drugs,
Cannot avert a summons that hath come.
What ails the physician that he dies of the disease
Which he used to cure in time gone by?
There died alike he who administered the drug, and he who took the drug,
And he who imported and sold the drug, and he who bought it."

Similar in purport are the following verses from the popular romance of 'Antara, the old Bedouin hero:

يقول لك الطبيب دواك عندى ‹   اذا ما جسّ زندك و الذراعا ‹

و لو علمِ الطبيب دوآهٖ دآءٍ ‹   يَرُدُّ الموت ما قاسى النزاعا ‹

" *The physician says to thee, 'I can cure thee,'*
When he feels thy wrist and thy arm;
But did the physician know a cure for disease
Which would ward off death, he would not himself suffer the death
  agony."

Now in considering the genesis and development
of the so-called Arabian Medicine, of which, though the
main outlines are clearly determined, many details
remain to be filled in, we may most conveniently begin
by enquiring what was the state of medical knowledge,
or ignorance, amongst the ancient Arabs before the
driving force of Islám destroyed their secular isolation,
sent them out to conquer half the then known world,
and brought this primitive but quick-witted people into
close contact with the ancient civilization of the Greeks,
Persians, Egyptians, Indians and others. We have to
distinguish three periods antecedent to what I have called
the Golden Age, viz.:

(1) The *Jáhiliyyat*, or Pagan Period, preceding the
rise and speedy triumph of Islám, which was fully
accomplished by the middle of the seventh century of
our era.

(2) The theocratic period of the Prophet and his
immediate successors, the Four Orthodox Caliphs, which
endured in all, from the *hijra* or "Flight" to the
assassination of 'Alí, less than forty years (A.D. 622–
661) and which had its centre at al-Madína, the ancient
Yathrib ('Ιάθριππα).

(3) The period of the Umayyad Caliphs, whose
immense Empire stretched from Spain to Samarqand,
and whose court at Damascus speedily began to show

a luxury and wealth hitherto utterly undreamed of by the Arabs.

For our present purpose it is hardly necessary to consider separately the first and second of these three periods, those namely which preceded and immediately followed the rise of Islám, and which, however widely they differed in their theological, ethical and political aspects, were, as regards scientific knowledge, almost on the same level. The life of the old pagan Arabs was rough and primitive in the highest degree—very much what the life of the Bedouin of Inner Arabia remains to this day;—the different tribes were constantly engaged in savage wars fomented by interminable vendettas; only the strong and resourceful could hold their own, and for the weak and sick there was little chance of survival. On the other hand they were intelligent, resourceful, courageous, hardy, chivalrous in many respects, very observant of all natural phenomena which came within the range of their observation, and possessed of a language of great wealth and virility of which they were inordinately proud, so that to this day, when they still praise God "who created the Arabic language the best of all languages," the poems of that far-off time, describing their raids, their battles, their venturous journeys and their love affairs, remain the standard and model of the chastest and most classical Arabic. Most of these warring tribes acknowledged no authority save that of their own chiefs and princes; only on the borders of the Persian and Roman Empires respectively, in the little kingdoms of Hira and Ghassán, did the elements of civilization and science exist.

The first Arab doctor mentioned by those careful biographers of philosophers and physicians, al-Qiftí and Ibn Abí Usaybi'a, is al-Hárith ibn Kalada, an elder contemporary of the Prophet Muḥammad, who had completed his studies at the great Persian medical school of Jundí-Shápúr, and who had the honour of being consulted on at least one occasion by the great Persian King Khusraw Anúsharwán (the Kisrá of the Arabs and Chosroes of the Greeks) who harboured and protected the Neo-Platonist philosophers driven into exile by the intolerance of the Emperor Justinian. An account of this interview, authentic or otherwise, fills a couple of closely-printed pages of Arabic in Ibn Abí Uṣaybi'a's *Classes of Physicians*, and the substance of it is given by Dr Lucien Leclerc in his *Histoire de la Médecine Arabe*. It consists almost entirely of general hygienic principles, sound enough as far as they go, but of little technical interest. A certain tragic interest attaches to Naḍr, the son of this al-Ḥárith[1], who like his father seems to have had some skill in medicine and a Persian education. This led him to mock at the biblical anecdotes contained in the *Qur'án*, these being, he did not hesitate to say, much less entertaining and instructive than the old Persian legends about Rustam and Isfandiyár, with which he would distract the attention and divert the interest of the Prophet's audience. Muḥammad never forgave him for this, and when he was taken prisoner at the Battle of Badr—the first notable victory of the Muslims over the unbelievers—he caused him to be put to death.

Of the Prophet's own ideas about medicine and

---

[1] My learned friend Mírzá Muḥammad of Qazwín, after reading these pages, has proved to me by many arguments and citations that Naḍr was not, as Ibn Abí Uṣaybi'a asserts, a son of al-Ḥárith ibn Kalada, the physician, of the tribe of Thaqíf, but of al-Ḥárith ibn 'Alqama ibn Kalada, a totally different person, though contemporary.

hygiene (partly derived, very likely, from the above-mentioned al-Ḥárith) we can form a fairly accurate idea from the very full and carefully authenticated body of traditions of his sayings and doings which, after the *Qur'án*, forms the most authoritative basis of Muhammadan doctrine. These traditions, finally collected and arranged during the ninth and tenth centuries of our era, are grouped according to subjects, each subject constituting a "book" (*kitáb*) and each tradition a "chapter" (*báb*). If we take the *Ṣaḥíḥ* of al-Bukhárí, the most celebrated of these collections, we find at the beginning of the fourth volume two books dealing with medicine and the sick, containing in all 80 chapters. This looks promising; but when we come to examine them more closely we find that only a small proportion deal with medicine, surgery or therapeutics as we understand them, and that the majority are concerned with such matters as the visitation, encouragement and spiritual consolation of the sick, the evil eye, magic, talismans, amulets and protective prayers and formulae. Although the Prophet declares that for every malady wherewith God afflicts mankind He has appointed a suitable remedy, he subsequently limits the principal methods of treatment to three, the administration of honey, cupping, and the actual cautery, and he recommends his followers to avoid or make sparing use of the latter. Camel's milk, fennel-flower (*Nigella sativa*), aloes, antimony (for ophthalmia), manna, and, as a styptic, the ashes of burnt matting, are amongst the other therapeutical agents mentioned. The diseases referred to include headache and migraine, ophthalmia, leprosy, pleurisy, pestilence and fever, which is characterized as "an exhalation of Hell." The Prophet advises his followers not to visit a country where pestilence

is raging, but not to flee from it if they find themselves
there. The scanty material furnished by these and other
traditions (for the *Qur'án*, apart from some mention of
wounds and a vague popular Embryology, contains
hardly any medical matter) has been more or less
systematized by later writers as what is termed *Ṭibbu'n-
Nabí*, or the "Prophet's Medicine," and I am informed
that a manual so entitled is still one of the first books
read by the student of the Old Medicine in India, along
with the abridgment of Avicenna's *Qánún* known as
the *Qánúncha*.

The ingenious Ibn Khaldún, whom we have already
had occasion to mention, speaks slightingly[1] of this
"Prophetic Medicine" and of the indigenous Arab
Medicine which it summarized and of which it formed
part, but judiciously adds that we are not called upon
to conform to its rules, since "the Prophet's mission
was to make known to us the prescriptions of the Divine
Law, and not to instruct us in Medicine and the common
practices of ordinary life." *À propos* of this he reminds
us that on one occasion the Prophet endeavoured to
forbid the artificial fecundation of the date-palm, with
such disastrous results to the fruit-crop that he with-
drew his prohibition with the remark, "You know
better than I do what concerns your worldly interests."
"One is then under no obligation," continues our author,
"to believe that the medical prescriptions handed down
even in authentic traditions have been transmitted to
us as rules which we are bound to observe; nothing in
these traditions indicates that this is the case. It is
however true that if one likes to employ these remedies
with the object of earning the Divine Blessing, and if
one takes them with sincere faith, one may derive from

[1] De Slane's transl., iii, pp. 163–4.

them great advantage, though they form no part of Medicine properly so-called."

I hope I have now said enough to show how wide was the difference between what passed for medical knowledge amongst the early Arabs of the pagan, prophetic and patriarchal periods, and the elaborate system built up on a Hippocratic and Galenic basis at Baghdád under the early 'Abbásid Caliphs. The facts here are certain and the data ample. More difficult is the question how far this system of Medicine was evolved under the Umayyad Caliphs in the intermediate period which lay between the middle of the seventh and the middle of the eighth centuries of the Christian era. These Umayyads, though, indeed, purely Arab, were by this time accustomed to the settled life and the amenities of civilization, and already far removed from the conquerors of Ctesiphon, the Sásánian capital, who mistook camphor for salt and found it insipid in their food; exchanged gold for an equal amount of silver— "the yellow for the white," as they expressed it;—and sold an incomparable royal jewel for a thousand pieces of money, because, as the vendor said when reproached for selling it so cheap, he knew no number beyond a thousand to ask for. Under these Umayyads the Arabian or Islamic Empire attained its maximum extent, for Spain, one of their chief glories, never acknowledged the 'Abbásid rule. In Egypt and Persia, as well as in Syria and its capital Damascus, where they held their court, they were in immediate contact with the chief centres of ancient learning. How far, we must enquire, did they profit by the opportunities thus afforded them ?

In the development of their theology, as von Kremer has shown[1], they were almost certainly influenced by

---

[1] *Culturgeschichte d. Orients*, vol. ii, pp. 401 *et seqq.*

John of Damascus, entitled Chrysorrhoas, and named in Arabic Manṣúr, who enjoyed the favour of the first Umayyad Caliph Mu'áwiya. The first impulse given to the desire of the Arabs for knowledge of the wisdom of the Greeks came from the Umayyad prince Khálid the son of Yazíd the son of Mu'áwiya, who had a passion for Alchemy. According to the *Fihrist*[1], the oldest and best existing source of our knowledge on these matters, he assembled the Greek philosophers in Egypt and commanded them to translate Greek and Egyptian books on this subject into Arabic; and these, says the author of the *Fihrist*, "were the first translations made in Islám from one language to another." With this prince is associated the celebrated Arabian alchemist Jábir ibn Ḥayyán, famous in medieval Europe under the name of Geber. Many, if not most, of the Latin books which passed under his name in the Middle Ages are spurious, being the original productions of European investigators who sought by the prestige attaching to his name to give authority and currency to their own writings. The Arabic originals of his works are rare, and the only serious study of them which I have met with is contained in the third volume of Berthelot's admirable *Histoire de la Chimie au Moyen Âge*, where the text and French translation of one of his genuine treatises are given. Berthelot points out, what, indeed, has long been recognized, that though the chief pursuit of the old alchemists was the Philosopher's Stone and the Elixir of Life, they nevertheless made many real and valuable discoveries. How many of these we owe to the Arabs is apparent in such words as *alcohol, alembic* and the like, still current amongst us. It is indeed generally recognized that it was in the domains of chemistry and

[1] p. 242.

materia medica that the Arabs added most to the body
of scientific doctrine which they inherited from the
Greeks.

Of medicine proper we find little trace amongst the
Arabs at this period, only three or four physicians being
specifically mentioned, mostly Christians, and probably
non-Arabs. One of them was Ibn Uthál, physician to
Mu'áwiya, the first Umayyad Caliph, who was murdered
by a man of the tribe of Makhzúm on suspicion of having,
at the instigation of the Caliph, poisoned an obnoxious
relative named 'Abdu'r-Rahmán. Another, Abu'l-
Hakam, also a Christian, lived to be a centenarian, as
did also his son Hakam. In the case of the latter we
have a fairly detailed account of his successful treatment
of a case of severe arterial haemorrhage caused by an
unskilful surgeon-barber. Neither of these men seems
to have written anything, but to 'Ísá the son of Hakam
is ascribed a large *Kunnásh*, or treatise on the Art of
Medicine, of which no fragment has been preserved.
Mention is also made by the Arab biographers of a certain Theodosius or Theodorus[1], evidently a Greek, who
was physician to the cruel but capable Hajjáj ibn Yúsuf,
by whom he was held in high honour and esteem. Some
of his aphorisms are preserved, but none of the three
or four works ascribed to him. The short list of these
medical practitioners of the Umayyad period is closed
by a Bedouin woman named Zaynab, who treated cases
of ophthalmia. That somewhat more attention began
to be paid to public health is indicated by the fact recorded by the historian Tabarí[2] that the Caliph al-Walíd
in the year 88/707 segregated the lepers, while as-

---

[1] Ibn Abí Usaybi'a (vol. i, pp. 121–123) gives the name in the
form of Thiyádhúq (ثیاذوق).

[2] Secunda Series, vol. ii, p. 1196.

signing to them an adequate supply of food. Amongst the Bedouin the recourse was still to the old charms and incantations, often accompanied by the application to the patient of the operator's saliva. An instance of this is recorded in connection with the poet Jarír[1], who gave his daughter Umm Ghaylán in marriage to a magician named Ablaq who had cured him in this fashion of erysipelas. The practice of medicine amongst the genuine Arabs of Arabia, both Bedouin and dwellers in towns, at the present day is succinctly described by Zwemer in his book *Arabia, the Cradle of Islám*[2]; and his description, so far as we can judge, fairly represents its condition at the remote period of which we are now speaking.

One important question demands consideration before we pass on to the great revival of learning under the early 'Abbásid Caliphs at Baghdád in the eighth and ninth centuries of our era. Leclerc in his *Histoire de la Médecine Arabe* maintains that already, a century earlier, when the Arabs conquered Egypt, the process of assimilating Greek learning began. In this process he assigns an important part to a certain Yaḥyá an-Naḥwí, or "John the Grammarian," who enjoyed high favour with 'Amr ibnu'l-'Áṣ, the conqueror and first Muslim governor of Egypt, and whom he identifies with John Philoponus the commentator of Aristotle. This Yaḥyá, of whom the fullest notice occurs in al-Qifṭí's "History of the Philosophers" (*Ta'ríkhu'l-Ḥukamá*)[3], was a Jacobite bishop at Alexandria, who subsequently repudiated the doctrine of the Trinity, and consequently attracted the favourable notice of the Muslims, to whose strict monotheism this doctrine is particularly obnoxious.

[1] Bevan's ed. of the *Naqá'iḍ*, p. 840.
[2] pp. 280–4. [3] Ed. Lippert, pp. 354–7.

He it was, according to the well-known story, now generally discredited by Orientalists, who was the ultimate though innocent cause of the alleged burning of the books in the great library at Alexandria by the Muslims, a story which Leclerc, in spite of his strong pro-Arab and pro-Muhammadan sympathies, oddly enough accepts as a historical fact[1]. This Yaḥyá, at any rate, was a great Greek scholar, and is said by al-Qifṭí to have mentioned in one of his works the year 343 of Diocletian (reckoned from A.D. 284) as the current year in which he wrote. This would agree very well with his presence in Egypt at the time of the Arab conquest in A.D. 640, but would prove that he was not identical with John Philoponus, who, according to a note added by Professor Bury to Gibbon's narrative of the event in question, flourished not in the seventh but in the early part of the sixth century after Christ[2]. The precious library of Alexandria had, as Gibbon observes, been pretty thoroughly destroyed by Christian fanatics nearly three centuries before the Muslims over-ran Egypt.

The questions of the fate of the Alexandrian library and the identity of the two Johns or Yaḥyás are, however, quite subordinate to the much larger and more important question of the state of learning in Egypt at the time of the Arab conquest. Leclerc's view is that the School of Medicine, once so famous, long outlived that of Philosophy, and continued, even though much fallen from its ancient splendour, until the time of the

---

[1] The arguments against the truth of this story are well set forth by L. Krehl (*Über die Sage von der Verbrennung der Alexandrinischen Bibliothek durch die Araber*) in the Acts of the Fourth International Congress of Orientalists (Florence, 1880).

[2] Vol. v of Bury's ed., p. 452 *ad calc.*

Arab conquest. This is a difficult point to decide; but Dr Wallis Budge, whose opinion I sought, definitely took the view that the Egyptian writings of this period at any rate, so far as they touched on these topics at all, showed little or no trace of medical science, Greek or other. At the same time we must give due weight to the well-authenticated Arabian tradition as to the translation of Greek works on Alchemy for the Umayyad prince Khálid ibn Yazíd in Egypt, and must admit the possibility, if not the probability, that these translations included other subjects, philosophical, medical and the like, besides that which constituted the aforesaid prince's special hobby.

Be this as it may, it was in the middle of the eighth century of our era and through the then newly-founded city of Baghdád that the great stream of Greek and other ancient learning began to pour into the Muhammadan world and to reclothe itself in an Arabian dress. And so far as Medicine is concerned, the tradition of the old Sásánian school of Jundí-Shápúr was predominant. Of this once celebrated school, now long a mere name, with difficulty located by modern travellers and scholars on the site of the hamlet of Sháh-ábád[1] in the province of Khúzistán in S.W. Persia, a brief account must now be given.

The city owed its foundation to the Sásánian monarch Shápúr I, the son and successor of Ardashír Bábakán who founded this great dynasty in the third century after Christ, and restored, after five centuries and a half of eclipse, the ancient glories of Achaemenian

---

[1] See Rawlinson's *Notes on a March from Zoháb to Khúzistán* in the *Journal of the Royal Geographical Society*, vol. ix, pp. 71–2, and Layard's remarks in vol. xvi, p. 86 of the same Journal.

Persia. Shápúr, after he had defeated and taken captive the Emperor Valerian, and sacked the famous city of Antioch, built, at the place called in Syriac Bêth Lâpât, a town which he named *Veh-az-Andev-i-Shápúr*, or "Shápúr's 'Better than Antioch,'" a name which was gradually converted into *Gundê Shápúr* or in Arabic *Jundí Sábúr*[1]. Another "Better than Antioch" was founded in the sixth century of our era by Khusraw Anúsharwán, the Chosroes of the Greeks and Kisrá of the Arabs, which, to distinguish it from the first, was called *Veh-az-Andev-i-Khusraw*. This latter town, by a practice which prevailed in Persia even until the sixteenth century, was chiefly populated by the deported citizens—especially craftsmen and artisans—of the foreign town after which it was named; and it seems likely that Jundí-Shápúr also received a considerable number of Greek settlers, for the Greek translations of Shápúr's Pahlawí inscriptions carved on the rocks at Istakhr in Fárs prove that Greek labour was available at this time even in the interior of Persia. Forty or fifty years later, in the early part of the fourth century, in the reign of the second Shápúr, the city had become a royal residence, and it was there that Mání or Manes, the founder of the Manichaean heresy, was put to death, and his skin, stuffed with straw, suspended from one of the city gates, known long afterwards, even in Muhammadan times, as the "Gate of Manes." There also, as appears probable, Shápúr II established the Greek physician Theodosius or Theodorus whom he summoned to attend him, and whose system of medicine is mentioned in the *Fihrist*[2] as one of the Persian books on Medicine after-

---

[1] See Th. Nöldeke's *Gesch. d. Perser u. Arab. zur Zeit der Sasaniden* (Leyden, 1879), pp. 40–42.

[2] p. 303.

wards translated into Arabic and preserved at any rate until the tenth century of our era. This physician, who was a Christian, obtained such honour and consideration in Persia that Shápúr caused a church to be built for him and at his request set free a number of his captive countrymen.

The great development of the school of Jundí-Shápúr was, however, the unforeseen and unintended result of that Byzantine intolerance which in the fifth century of our era drove the Nestorians from their school at Edessa and forced them to seek refuge in Persian territory. In the following century the enlightened and wisdom-loving Khusraw Anúsharwán, the protector of the exiled Neo-Platonist philosophers[1], sent his physician Burzúya to India, who, together with the game of chess and the celebrated *Book of Kalíla and Dimna*, brought back Indian works on medicine and also, apparently, Indian physicians to Persia.

The school of Jundí-Shápúr was, then, at the time of the Prophet Muḥammad's birth, at the height of its glory. There converged Greek and Oriental learning, the former transmitted in part directly through Greek scholars, but for the most part through the industrious and assimilative Syrians, who made up in diligence what they lacked in originality. Sergius of Ra'su'l-'Ayn, who flourished a little before this time[2], was one of those who translated Hippocrates and Galen into Syriac. Of this intermediate Syriac medical literature, from which many, perhaps most, of the Arabic translations of the eighth and ninth centuries were made, not much survives, but M. H. Pognon's edition and French translation of a Syriac version of the *Aphorisms*[3] of Hippocrates, and

---

[1] About A.D. 531. [2] He died at Constantinople about A.D. 536.
[3] *Une Version Syriaque des Aphorismes d'Hippocrate*, Leipzig, 1903.

BAM 3

Dr Wallis Budge's *Syriac Book of Medicines*[1], enable us to form some idea of its quality. To the Syrians, whatever their defects, and especially to the Nestorians, Asia owes much, and the written characters of the Mongol, Manchu, Úyghúr and many other peoples in the western half of Asia testify to the literary influence of the Aramaic peoples.

But though the medical teaching of Jundí-Shápúr was in the main Greek, there was no doubt an underlying Persian element, especially in Pharmacology, where the Arabic nomenclature plainly reveals in many cases Persian origins. Unfortunately the two most glorious periods of pre-Islamic Persia, the Achaemenian (B.C. 550–330) and the Sásánian (A.D. 226–640) both terminated in a disastrous foreign invasion, Greek in the first case, Arab in the second, which involved the wholesale destruction of the indigenous learning and literature, so that it is impossible for us to reconstitute more than the main outlines of these two ancient civilizations. Yet the *Avesta*, the sacred book of the Zoroastrians, speaks of three classes of healers, by prayers and religious observances, by diet and drugs, and by instruments; in other words priests, physicians and surgeons. As regards the latter, one curious passage in the *Vendîdâd* ordains that the tyro must operate successfully on three unbelievers before he may attempt an operation on one of the "good Mazdayasnian religion." And, of course, Greek physicians, of whom Ctesias is the best known, besides an occasional Egyptian, were to be found at the Achaemenian court before the time of Alexander of Macedon.

The medical school of Jundí-Shápúr seems to have been little affected by the Arab invasion and conquest

---

[1] Two vols., text and translation, 1913.

of the seventh century of our era, but it was not till the latter half of the eighth century, when Baghdád became the metropolis of Islám, that its influence began to be widely exerted on the Muslims. It was in the year A.D. 765[1] that the second 'Abbásid Caliph al-Manṣúr, being afflicted with an illness which baffled his medical advisers, summoned to attend him Júrjís the son of Bukht-Yishú'(a half-Persian, half-Syriac name, meaning "Jesus hath delivered")[2], the chief physician of the great hospital of Jundí-Shápúr. Four years later Júrjís fell ill and craved permission to return home, to see his family and children, and, should he die, to be buried with his fathers. The Caliph invited him to embrace the religion of Islám, but Júrjís replied that he preferred to be with his fathers, whether in heaven or hell. Thereat the Caliph laughed and said, "Since I saw thee I have found relief from the maladies to which I had been accustomed," and he dismissed him with a gift of 10,000 *dínárs*, and sent with him on his journey an attendant who should convey him, living or dead, to Jundí-Shápúr, the "Civitas Hippocratica" which he loved so well. Júrjís on his part promised to send to Baghdád to replace him one of his pupils named 'Ísá ibn Shahlá, but declined to send his son, Bukht-Yishú' the second, on the ground that he could not be spared from the *Bímáristán*, or hospital, of Jundí-Shápúr.

For six generations and over 250 years the Bukht-Yishú' family remained pre-eminent in medicine, the last (Jibrá'íl son of 'Ubaydu'lláh son of Bukht-Yishú' son of Jibrá'íl son of Bukht-Yishú' son of Júrjís son of

---

[1] Al-Qifṭí's *Ta'ríkhu'l-Ḥukamá*, p. 158.

[2] The explanation of these old Persian names beginning or ending with *-bukht* we owe to Professor Th. Nöldeke, *Gesch. d. Artakhshír-i-Pápakán*, p. 49, n. 4.

Jibrá'íl), who died on April 10, 1006, being as eminent and as highly honoured by the rulers and nobles of his time as the first. That a certain exclusiveness and un-willingness to impart their knowledge to strangers charac-terized the physicians of Jundí-Shápúr may be inferred from the treatment received at the beginning of his career by the celebrated tranślator of Greek medical works into Arabic, Ḥunayn ibn Isḥáq, known to medi-eval Europe as "Johannitius." He was a Christian of Ḥíra with a great passion for knowledge, and acted as dispenser to Yuḥanná ibn Másawayh (the "Messues" of the Latino-Barbari), whose lectures he also followed. But he was prone to ask too many troublesome questions, and one day his master, losing patience, exclaimed, "What have the people of Ḥíra to do with medicine? Go and change money in the streets!" and drove him forth in tears; "for," says al-Qifṭí[1], "these people of Jundí-Shápúr used to believe that they only were worthy of this science, and would not suffer it to go forth from themselves, their children and their kin." But Ḥunayn, more resolved than ever on pursuing knowledge to its source, went away for several years to learn Greek. During this period one of his former acquaintances, Yúsuf the physician, one day saw a man with long hair and unclipped beard and moustaches reciting Homer in the street, and, in spite of his changed appearance, recognized his voice as that of Ḥunayn. He, being questioned, admitted his identity, but enjoined silence on Yúsuf, saying that he had sworn not to continue his medical studies until he had perfected himself in know-ledge of the Greek language. When he finally returned, Jibrá'íl ibn Bukht-Yishú', to whom he attached himself, was delighted with his Greek scholarship and declared

[1] *Op. cit.*, p. 174.

him to be a miracle of learning, and Ibn Másawayh, who had formerly driven him out with contumely, sought Yúsuf's good offices to effect a reconciliation with him. Later he gained high favour with the Caliph, who, however, was minded first to prove his professional honour by a hard test, for he bade him concoct a poison for one of his enemies, offering him rich rewards if he would do so, but severe punishment—imprisonment or death—if he refused. He refused and was imprisoned for a year, when he was again brought before the Caliph and bidden to choose again between compliance and a rich reward, or the sword of the executioner. " I have already told the Commander of the Faithful," replied Ḥunayn, "that I have skill only in what is beneficial, and have studied naught else"; and being again threatened with instant death he added, " I have a Lord who will give me my right to-morrow in the Supreme Uprising, so if the Caliph would injure his own soul, let him do so." Then the Caliph smiled and declared that he had only desired to assure himself of Ḥunayn's probity before yielding him implicit confidence. So the incident ended satisfactorily, but it serves to show that the position of Court Physician at Baghdád in early 'Abbásid times was sometimes a trying one ; a fact brought out in the well-known story of the physician Dúbán and King Yúnán (which, however, had a much more tragic ending) in the *Arabian Nights*[1].

Ḥunayn was not only the most celebrated but the most productive of these translators. Of the ten Hippocratic writings mentioned by the author of the *Fihrist* as existing in Arabic translations in his time, seven were his work and three the work of his pupil 'Ísá ibn Yaḥyá, while the "sixteen books" of Galen were all translated by

[1] Lane's translation (London, 1859), vol. i, pp. 83–6.

him or his pupil Ḥubaysh. Generally, as we learn from the *Fihrist*[1], Ḥunayn translated the Greek into Syriac, while Hubaysh translated from Syriac into Arabic, the Arabic version being then revised by Ḥunayn, who, however, sometimes translated directly from Greek into Arabic. All three languages were known to most of these translators, and it is probable, as Leclerc suggests, that whether the translation was made into Syriac or Arabic depended on whether it was primarily designed for Christian or Muslim readers. At the present day comparatively few of these Arabic translations are available, even in manuscript; but good MSS. of the *Aphorisms*[2] and *Prognostics*[3] exist in the British Museum, besides an epitome of the "sixteen books" of Galen[4] ascribed to Yaḥyá an-Naḥwí, or "John the Grammarian." Of the *Aphorisms* in Arabic there is an Indian lithographed edition, which, however, I have not seen. This dearth of texts is very unfortunate for the student of Arabian Medicine, who is thereby much hampered in the solution of two important preliminary questions, viz. the accuracy and fidelity of these early Arabic translations, and the development of the Arabic medical terminology, often unintelligible without reference to the Greek original. As regards the first question, Leclerc[5] is apparently right in his opinion that the translation from Greek into Arabic was generally effected with much greater skill and knowledge than the later translation from Arabic into Latin, and that he who judges Arabian Medicine only by the latter will inevitably undervalue it and do it a great injustice. Indeed it is difficult

---

[1] p. 289.
[2] Or. 5914, Or. 6419, Or. 5820, Or. 6386, and Or. 5939.
[3] Or. 5914.   [4] Arundel, Or. 17.
[5] *Hist. de la Médecine Arabe*, vol. ii, pp. 346–8.

to resist the conclusion that many passages in the Latin version of the *Qánún* of Avicenna were misunderstood or not understood at all by the translator, and consequently can never have conveyed a clear idea to the reader. Another group of great translators from Greek into Arabic was provided by the city of Ḥarrán, the classical Charrae, which remained pagan down to the thirteenth century, and, by reason of the high degree of Greek culture long maintained there, was known as Hellenopolis. How the inhabitants of this city came to be known as "Sabaeans" from the ninth century onwards, though they had nothing to do with the true Sabaeans of Chaldaea (of whom a remnant, known to the Muhammadans as *al-Mughtasila* from their frequent ceremonial bathings and washings, and to Europeans, for the same reason, as "Christians of St John the Baptist," exist to the present day near Baṣra and along the banks of the Shaṭṭu'l-'Arab), is a very curious story, exhaustively set forth, with full documentary evidence, by Chwolson in his great work *Die Ssabier und Ssabismus*[1]. Of these learned Ḥarránians the most celebrated were Thábit ibn Qurra (born A.D. 836, died A.D. 901), his sons Ibráhím and Sinán, his grandsons Thábit and Ibráhím, and his great-grandson Sinán; and the family of Zahrún. Mention should also be made of another contemporary translator, though his predilection was for mathematics rather than medicine, Qusṭá ibn Lúqá, a Christian of Baalbek in Syria, who died about A.D. 923.

Thus by the tenth century the Muslims, to all of whom, irrespective of race, Arabic was not only the language of Revelation and Religion, but also of science, diplomacy and polite intercourse, had at their disposal

[1] St Petersburg, 1856 (2 vols.). See vol. i, ch. vi (pp. 139–157).

a great mass of generally excellent translations of all
the most famous philosophical and scientific writings of
the Greeks. For Greek poetry and drama they cared
little, and of the Latin writers they seem to have known
nothing whatever. Of the Greek medical writers, besides
Hippocrates and Galen, their favourites were Rufus of
Ephesus, Oribasius, Paul of Ægina, and Alexander of
Tralles; and, for materia medica, Dioscorides. In some
cases Greek writings, lost in the original, have been preserved to us in Arabic translations. The most notable
instance of this is afforded by the seven books of Galen's
Anatomy (ix–xv), lost in the original Greek but preserved in the Arabic, of which the text, with German
translation and full *apparatus criticus*, has been published
by Dr Max Simon[1], with an admirable Arabic-Greek-
German vocabulary of technical terms, to which reference has already been made.

Were the materials accessible, it would be interesting
to compare those Arabic translations made directly from
the Greek with those which first passed through the
medium of Syriac. Of the few Syriac versions preserved
to us I cannot myself form an opinion, being unfortunately unacquainted with that language, but they are
rather harshly judged by M. Pognon, of whose edition
and translation of the Syriac *Aphorisms* of Hippocrates
I have already spoken[2]. "The Syriac version of the
Aphorisms contained in my manuscript," he writes,
"is a very faithful, or rather too faithful, translation of
the Greek text; sometimes, indeed, it is a literal translation absolutely devoid of sense. This, unfortunately,
does not allow us to determine the epoch at which it

---

[1] *Sieben Bücher Anatomie des Galen, u.s.w.*, 2 vols. (Leipzig, 1906).

[2] *Une Version Syriaque des Aphorismes d'Hippocrate, texte et tra-
duction, par M. Pognon, Consul de France à Alep* (Leipzig, 1903).

was made, since to render too literally has been the defect of many Syrian translators."

"I will not venture to say," he continues, "that the Syrians never possessed clear translations written in a correct style, but in most of the translations which have reached us the style is often obscure, the construction incorrect, and words are often employed in a sense not properly belonging to them, this generally arising from the desire of the Syriac translator to reproduce the Greek text too faithfully. The Syrian translators, when they found a difficult passage, too often contented themselves with rendering each Greek word by a Syriac word without in any way seeking to write an intelligible sentence. Thus we find in their translations many incorrect sentences, and even expressions which have absolutely no meaning. In short, I believe that when they did not understand the meaning of a Greek word, the translators did not hesitate to transcribe it in Syriac characters, leaving their readers to conjecture the meaning of these barbarisms which they had created." The translation of the *Aphorisms*, with which he is specially concerned, M. Pognon characterizes as "detestable," and adds: "Whenever the translator comes across an obscure passage, his translation is obscure; and whenever he meets with a passage which is susceptible of several different renderings, his translation can be interpreted in several different ways." This assertion he proves by numerous examples.

The Arab mind, on the other hand, is clear and positive, and the Arabic language nervous, virile and rich both actually and potentially. The old Arabs were an acute and observant people, and for all natural objects which fell under their notice they had appropriate and finely differentiated words. To render the medical

works of the Greeks into their own language they had,
of course, in many cases, to invent new terms translated
or imitated from the Greek, and often only to be understood by reference to the Greek originals; but they
already possessed a fairly copious anatomical vocabulary,
which, moreover, they were fond of using in ordinary
life, even in their poetry. Thus the Umayyad Caliph
Yazíd ibn 'Abdu'l-Malik, who, in 105/723–4, died of
love for the slave-girl Ḥabbába, was deeply stirred by
her singing of the following verse[1]:

بَيْنَ ٱلتَّرَاقِى وَ ٱللَّهَاةِ حَرَارَةٌ * مَا تَطْمَئِنُّ وَ لاَ تَسُوغُ فَتَبْرُدُ،

*"Between the clavicles and the uvula is a burning heat
Which cannot be appeased or swallowed down and cooled."*

The poet al-Mutanabbí (tenth century) has a poem[2]
on a fever by which he was attacked in Egypt in
Dhu'l-Ḥijja 348 (February 960), and which left him—

عليلُ الجسمِ ممتنعُ القيامِ * شديدُ السُّكْرِ من غيرِ ٱلمُدامِ،

"Sick of body, unable to rise up, vehemently intoxicated (i.e. delirious)
without wine."

He compares the fever to a coy maiden who will
only visit him under cover of darkness:

فليس تزور آلّا فى الظَّلامِ،	و زائرتى كأنَّ بها حياءً،
فعافَتْها و باتَتْ فى عِظَامى،	بذلْتُ لها المطارف و الحشايا،
فتُوسِعُهُ بأنواع السَّقامِ،	يضيق الجلْدُ عن نَفَسى وعنها،
كأنّا عاكفانِ على حرامِ،	اذا ما فارقَتْنى غسَّلْتْنى،
مدامعها بأربعة سجامِ،	كأنّ الصُّبْحَ يَطْرُدُهَا فتجرى،

[1] *Kitábu 'l-Fakhrí*, ed. Ahlwardt, p. 155.
[2] Ed. Dieterici, pp. 675–680.

أُراقِب وقتها من غير شوقٍ،   مراقبة المشوق المستهامِ،

و يَصْدُقُ وَعْدُهَا و الصّدق شرٌّ،   اذا أَلقاك فى الكُرَب العظامِ،

"And it is as though she who visits me were filled with modesty,
For she does not pay her visits save under cover of darkness.
I freely offered her my linen and my pillows,
But she refused them, and spent the night in my bones.
My skin is too contracted to contain both my breath and her,
So she relaxes it with all sorts of sickness.
When she leaves me, she washes me [with perspiration]
As though we had retired apart for some forbidden action.
It is as though the morning drives her away,
And her lachrymal ducts are flooded in their four channels.
I watch for her time [of arrival] without desire,
Yet with the watchfulness of the eager lover.
And she is ever faithful to her appointed time, but faithfulness is an evil
When it casts thee into grievous sufferings."

Under such astonishing imagery are clearly depicted the delirium and regular nightly recurrence of the fever, the rigors which mark its onset, and the copious perspiration with which it concludes, the latter being fantastically likened to the weeping of a woman torn from her lover's arms.

That in the days of the Caliphate every educated person was expected to take some interest in Medicine and to know something about Anatomy is shown by the curious story of the equally fair and talented slave-girl Tawaddud in the *Arabian Nights*. The girl is offered to the Caliph Hárúnu'r-Rashíd for an enormous price (10,000 *dínárs*) by her bankrupt master Abu'l-Ḥusn, and the Caliph agrees to pay this sum provided she can answer satisfactorily any questions addressed to her by those most learned in each of the many branches of knowledge in which she claims to excel. Therefore the most notable professors of Theology, Law, Exegesis of the *Qur'án*, Medicine, Astronomy, Philosophy, Rhetoric and Chess examine her in succession, and in each case she not only gives satisfactory replies to all their questions, but ends by putting to each of them a question which he is unable to answer. Lane describes this story, which provides material for six of the 1001 Nights[1], as "extremely tiresome to most readers," but it is very valuable as indicating what was regarded by the medieval Muslims as a good all-round education. The medical portion of the examination includes the outlines of Anatomy and Physiology, according to Arabian ideas, diagnosis from signs and symptoms, humoristic Pathology, Hygiene, Dietetics and the like. The enumeration of the bones is fairly complete, but that of the blood-vessels very vague. Of the branches of the Aorta, says Tawaddud, "none knoweth the tale save He who created them, but it is said that they number 360"—a mystical number, 12 × 30, which still plays a great part in the doctrines of certain Muhammadan sects, by whom it is called "The Number of All Things" (عدد كل شئ) for reasons which it would be tedious to enumerate in this place.

I have already taken up too much of your time this afternoon in the discussion of these preliminaries. In my next lecture I propose to speak of four of the most notable early medical writers of the Muslims who succeeded the epoch of the great translators. These were all Persians by race, though they wrote in Arabic; and the Latin versions of the chief works of three of them, known to the Latino-Barbari as Rhazes, Haly Abbas and Avicenna, constituted three of the most highly esteemed medical works current in medieval Europe.

[1] Nights 449–454; ed. Macnaghten, vol. ii, pp. 512–521; Sir R. Burton's translation, vol. v, pp. 218–227.

LECTURE II

In my last lecture I traced the growth of the so-called "Arabian Medicine" down to the ninth century of our era, the time of the great translators of the early 'Abbásid period; and I showed how, by their diligence and learning, the teachings of the most eminent physicians of Ancient Greece, notably Hippocrates, Galen, Oribasius, Rufus of Ephesus and Paul of Ægina, were rendered accessible to the Muslim world. We must now pass to the independent Arabic writers on medicine, who, starting from this foundation, compiled more or less original works embodying, to some extent, observations of their own, and arranged on their own plan. The great extent of the subject, however, obliges me to impose on myself somewhat strict limitations of region, period and topic, and I shall therefore confine myself to the two centuries immediately succeeding the Golden Age, which lies between A.D. 750 and 850, and to the Eastern lands of the Caliphate, especially Persia. Further, I shall confine myself to four or five of the principal medical writers of this limited period, and, as a rule, to one only of the works of each. Even under such limitations only a very partial and superficial view can be obtained, for a whole series of lectures might evidently be devoted to a single section of any one of the works which I propose briefly to discuss to-day.

Before proceeding further, however, there are one or two preliminary matters on which a few words should be said, and first of all as to the evolution of Arabic scientific terminology. The Syrians, as we have seen, were too much disposed to transcribe Greek words as they stood, without any attempt at elucidation, leaving the reader to make the best he could of them. The medieval Latin translators from the Arabic did exactly the same, and the Latin *Qánún* of Avicenna swarms with barbarous words which are not merely transcriptions, but in many cases almost unrecognizable mistranscriptions, of Arabic originals. Thus the coccyx is named in Arabic *'uṣ'uṣ* (عُصْعُص), or, with the definite article, *al-'uṣ'uṣ* (ٱلْعُصْعُص), which appears in the Latin version as *alhosos*; *al-qaṭan* (ٱلقَطَن), the lumbar region, appears as *alchatim*; *al-'ajuz* or *al-'ajiz* (العجِز), the sacrum, variously appears as *alhauis* and *al-hagiazi*; and *an-nawájidh* (النّواجِذ), the wisdom-teeth, as *nuaged* or *neguegidi*. Dozens of similar monstrosities can be gleaned from Dr Hyrtl's *Das Arabische und Hebräische in der Anatomie* (Vienna, 1879), and it must be confessed that the Arabs also were, in a lesser degree, guilty of a similar mutilation of Greek words, as, for example, the transformation of ἀμνεῖος into *anfas* (أَنْفَس), which in turn, in the hands of the Latino-Barbari, became *abgas*.

Generally, however, in spite of the fact that the Arabic language almost entirely lacks the Greek facility of forming compound words to express new and complex ideas, the Arabs succeeded in paraphrasing the Greek technical terms with fair success. *Diagnosis* is fairly rendered by *tashkhíṣ*, which primarily means the identification of a person (*shakhṣ*); *prognosis* is more cumbrously rendered by *taqdimatu'l-ma'rifati*, literally, the sending forward of knowledge. In the earliest Arabic medical books, like the *Firdawsu'l-Ḥikmat*, or "Paradise of Wisdom," of which I shall speak immediately, strange Syro-Persian words, probably borrowed from the vocabulary of Jundí-Shápúr, and subsequently replaced by good Arabic equivalents, appear. Thus in the almost unique MS. of the work just mentioned there twice occurs a word for a headache affecting the whole head (as contrasted with *shaqíqa*, which denotes hemicrania or migraine), faultily written in both cases (once as سنوریا and once as سوریتا), which only after numerous enquiries of Syriac scholars was identified as the Syriac *sanwartả* (ܣܢܘܪܬܐ), said to be a Persian word meaning primarily a helmet. And in fact it is evidently the Persian *sar-band* (سَرْبَنْد) or *sar-wand* with transposition of the *r* and the *n* (*san-ward* for *sar-wand*) and the addition of the Syriac final emphatic *ả*. This may serve as an instance of the kind of trouble which the reader or translator, or still more the editor, of these old Arabic medical works is apt to meet with, for of scarcely any, even of the few which have been published in the original, do critical editions exist.

On the other hand, apart from the fairly copious anatomical, pathological and medical vocabulary properly belonging to the Arabic language, it has a great power of forming significant derivatives from existing rôots, which, when formed, are at once intelligible. Thus there exists in Arabic a special form for the "noun of pain," wherein the first root-letter is followed by a short *u* and the second by a long *ā* (the form known to Arab grammarians as فُعَال, *fuʿál*), and this is the form assumed by the names of most diseases and ailments; as the already mentioned *ṣudáʿ* (صُدَاع), "a splitting headache," the "*soda*" of the Latino-Barbari; *zukám* (زُكَام), "a catarrh"; *judhám* (جُذَام), "elephantiasis," etc. On this analogy we get, from the root *dawr* (دَوْر), "revolving," *duwár* (دُوَار), "vertigo," the sickness produced by being whirled round; from *baḥr* (بَحْر), "the sea," *buḥár* (بُحَار),

"sea-sickness"; from *khamr* (خَمْر); "wine," *khumár* (خُمَار), the headache resulting from undue indulgence in wine; and so forth. I never met with the word *jubál* (جُبَال) from *jabal* (جَبَل), "a mountain," but, if I did meet with it, I should know that it could mean nothing else but "mountain-sickness." In other cases the Arabic technical term implies a pathological theory, as, for example, *istisqá* (اِسْتِسْقَاء), *mustasqí* (مُسْتَسْقِى), which are respectively the verbal noun and the active participle of the tenth, or desiderative, conjugation of the root *saqa, yasqí* (سَقَى يَسْقِى), "to give drink to," and in ordinary language mean "craving for drink" and "one who craves for drink," but in Medicine "dropsy" and "dropsical," conformably to the familiar Latin adage, *Crescit indulgens sibi dirus hydrops.* Thus it will be apparent that Arabic is on the whole well adapted for providing a suitable technical terminology, which, in fact, it has done for the whole Muslim world, whether they speak Arabic, Persian, Turkish or Urdú, and which, as the modern Egyptian Press testifies, it continues to do at the present day.

Another point deserving brief notice is the question whether dissection was ever practised by the Muslims. The answer is usually given in the negative, and I must admit that I incline to this view; but in an immense, unfinished, modern Persian biographical dictionary entitled *Náma-ı-Dánishwarán,* "the Book of Learned Men," compiled by command of the late Náṣiru'd-Dín Sháh by four learned men, to wit Mírzá Abu'l-Faḍl of Sáwa the physician, Shaykh Muḥammad Mahdí 'Abdu'r-Rabb-ábádí, entitled *Shamsu'l-'Ulamá,* Mírzá Ḥasan-i-Ṭálaqání, entitled *Adíb,* and Mirzá 'Abdu'l-Wahháb ibn 'Abdu'l-'Alí of Qazwín, and lithographed at Ṭihrán

25 years ago, it is stated[1] that the celebrated Yuḥanná ibn Másawayh, being unable to obtain human subjects, dissected apes in a special dissecting-room which he built on the banks of the Tigris, and that a particular species of ape, considered to resemble man most closely, was, by command of the Caliph al-Muʻtaṣim, supplied to him about the year A.D. 836 by the ruler of Nubia. This story is given on the authority of Ibn Abí Uṣaybiʻa, in whose *Classes of Physicians*[2] it in fact occurs in a less clear and detailed form. It is, however, not to be found in al-Qiftí's *History of the Philosophers*, and cannot, I fear, be regarded as affording weighty evidence as to the practice of dissection in the medical schools of the Arabs. This Yuḥanná ibn Másawayh had a bad temper and a sharp tongue. According to the *Fihrist* he once said to a courtier who had annoyed him, "If the ignorance wherewith thou art afflicted were converted into understanding, and then divided amongst a hundred beetles, each one of them would be more sagacious than Aristotle!"

To come now to the medical writers of whom I propose to speak this afternoon, the oldest of them is ʻAlí ibn Rabban of Ṭabaristán, the Persian province south of the Caspian Sea. Rabban, as he himself explains at the beginning of his book, was the title, not the name, of his father.

"My father," he says, "was the son of a certain scribe of the city of Merv...who had a great zeal for the pursuit of virtue...and sought to derive benefit from books on Medicine and Philosophy, preferring Medicine to the profession of his fathers. Herein his object was not so much to seek after praise and profit as to conform himself to the Divine Attributes, and so to earn

[1] Vol. ii, pp. 37–8.   [2] Vol. i, p. 178 of the Cairo ed.

the consideration of mankind. Wherefore he received the title of *Rabban*, which being interpreted signifies 'our Master' and 'our Teacher.'"

From this title we may infer that our author's father was a Christian or a Jew, and in fact al-Qiftí[1], who gives a short notice of him, says that he professed the latter religion; that the father's proper name was Sahl, and that the son only made profession of Islám after he entered the service of the Caliph al-Mutawakkil. Previously to this he had been secretary to the celebrated Mázyár, of the noble Persian house of Qáren, who rebelled against the Caliph in the hope of liberating his country from the Arab yoke, and was finally captured and crucified at Baghdád beside the heresiarch Bábak. 'Alí ibn Rabban subsequently entered the service of the Caliph, and finally, in the third year of his reign (A.D. 850), succeeded, after many interruptions, in completing the work on Medicine and Natural Philosophy on which he had long been engaged, and which he entitled *Firdawsu'l-Ḥikmat*, the "Paradise of Wisdom." This is nearly all that is known of his life, except that from an illustration given in his book[2] it is evident that he was, as his *nisba* implies, familiar with the mountains and mists of Ṭabaristán, and the much more important fact that he was one of the teachers of the great physician ar-Rází or Rhazes, a fact which in itself invests his work with considerable interest. According to the *Fihrist*[3] he only wrote four books, of which the "Paradise of Wisdom" is the most important. It must at one time have been well known and highly esteemed, for, as we learn from Yáqút's *Dictionary of Learned Men*[4], the great historian Muḥammad ibn Jarír aṭ-

---

[1] p. 231.   [2] Brit. Mus. MS. **Arundel, Or. 41**, f. 15*a*.
[3] p. 296.   [4] "E. J. W. Gibb Memorial" Series, vi, 6, p. 429.

Tabarí was reading it while he lay sick in bed; while in another passage of the same work[1], where that eminent patron of letters the Ṣáḥib Isma'íl ibn 'Abbád is censured for imagining himself to be superior to all the greatest authorities in every science and art, the *Firdaws*, or "Paradise," of 'Alí ibn Rabban[2] is mentioned amongst those authorities. Subsequently this book, like so many other precious Arab works, became almost extinct, and at the present day, so far as I can ascertain, there exist only two manuscripts of it, one fine old copy (**Arundel, Or. 41**) in the British Museum, which I have had photographed for my use; and another (**Landberg, 266**) at Berlin; but this latter copy seems, so far as I have been able to learn, to be only an abridgment, or at least to contain a somewhat mutilated or abbreviated text.

The "Paradise of Wisdom," which I hope some day to edit and perhaps translate, deals chiefly with Medicine, but also to some extent with Philosophy, Meteorology, Zoology, Embryology, Psychology and Astronomy. It is a fair-sized book containing nearly 550 pages, and is divided into 7 parts (*Naw'*), 30 discourses (*Maqála*), and 360 chapters. The author mentions as his principal sources Hippocrates, Aristotle, Galen, Yuḥanná ibn Másawayh (Messues) and Ḥunayn "the Interpreter," *i.e.* Ḥunayn ibn Isḥáq, the medieval Johannitius. The fourth and last Discourse of the seventh Part contains in 36 chapters a summary of Indian Medicine. It would be tedious to you if I were to read out the abstract of the contents of the book which I have made, nor would the author himself have approved such a procedure, for he says:

" He who perpends this book with understanding

---

[1] "E. J. W. Gibb Memorial" Series, vi, 2, p. 279.
[2] The text erroneously has زين (*Zayn*) for ربن (*Rabban*).

resembles one who wanders in fruitful and pleasant gardens, or in the markets of great cities, wherein is provided for each of the senses its pleasure and delight. But just as he who limits his knowledge of such gardens and cities to the contemplation of their gates is as one who seeth naught of them, so he who enumerates the chapters of this my book without attentively reading what is contained in each, doth not understand the true meaning of what I say....But he who masters this book, and fully fathoms and perpends it, will find in it the greater part of what the young graduate needs of the Science of Medicine and the action of the natural forces in this Microcosm and also in the Macrocosm."

Some justification is perhaps needed for rendering the Arabic word *mutakharrij* in the above passage in its modern sense of "graduate," which may seem too definite a translation of a word implying one who comes out, or issues forth, from a school or college at which he has completed his studies. It is therefore worth noting that some sort of qualifying examination in medicine, if it did not already exist in A.D. 850, when our author wrote, was instituted 80 years later in the reign of the Caliph al-Muqtadir on account of a case of malpraxis which came to his notice in A.D. 931. He thereupon issued an order, as al-Qifṭí informs us[1], that none should practise medicine in Baghdád unless he was able to satisfy Sinán ibn Thábit of Ḥarrán of his competence and proficiency, with the exception of a few physicians of recognized standing, who, on account of their reputation, were exempted from this test, to which the remainder, numbering some 860, had to submit. That the examination was not always of a very searching character is shown by the following incident. Amongst

[1] *Ta'ríkhu'l-Ḥukamá*, pp. 191–2.

the practitioners who presented themselves before Sinán was a dignified and well-dressed old man of imposing appearance. Sinán accordingly treated him with consideration and respect, and addressed to him various remarks on the cases before him. When the other candidates had been dismissed, he said, " I should like to hear from the Shaykh (Professor) something which I may remember from him, and that he should mention who was his Teacher in the Profession." Thereupon the old gentleman laid a packet of money before Sinán and said, "I cannot read or write well, nor have I read anything systematically, but I have a family whom I maintain by my professional labours, which, therefore, I beg you not to interrupt." Sinán laughed and replied, "On condition that you do not treat any patient with what you know nothing about, and that you do not prescribe phlebotomy or any purgative drug save for simple ailments." "This," said the old man, "has been my practice all my life, nor have I ever ventured beyond *sirkangabín* (oxymel) and *julláb* (jalap)." Next day amongst those who presented themselves before Sinán was a well-dressed young man of pleasing and intelligent appearance. "With whom did you study?" enquired Sinán. "With my father," answered the youth. "And who is your father?" asked Sinán. "The old gentleman who was with you yesterday," replied the other. " A fine old gentleman!" exclaimed Sinán ; "and do you follow his methods ?...Yes ?...Then see to it that you do not go beyond them ! "

Although, as I have said, a detailed statement of the contents of the "Paradise of Wisdom" would be out of place, the general plan of the book may be briefly indicated.

PART I. Treats of certain general philosophical ideas, the categories, natures, elements, metamorphosis, genesis and decay.

PART II. Treats of embryology, pregnancy, the functions and morphology of different organs, ages and seasons, psychology, the external and internal senses, the temperaments and emotions, personal idiosyncrasies, certain nervous affections (tetanus, torpor, palpitation, nightmare, etc.), the evil eye, hygiene and dietetics.

PART III. Treats of nutrition and dietetics.

PART IV. (The longest, comprising 12 Discourses) treats of general and special pathology, from the head to the feet, and concludes with an account of the number of muscles, nerves and veins, and dissertations on phlebotomy, the pulse and urinoscopy.

PART V. Treats of tastes, scents and colours.

PART VI. Treats of materia medica and toxicology.

PART VII. Treats of climate, waters and seasons in their relation to health, outlines of cosmography and astronomy, and the utility of the science of medicine: and concludes, as already noted, with a summary of Indian Medicine in 36 chapters.

It will be noticed that the book contains very little about anatomy or surgery and a great deal about climate, diet and drugs, including poisons. Part IV, dealing with pathology, is on the whole the most interesting, and I may, perhaps, be permitted to enumerate more fully the contents of the 12 Discourses which it comprises:

Discourse 1 (9 chapters) on general pathology, the signs and symptoms of internal disorders, and the principles of therapeutics.

Discourse 2 (14 chapters) on diseases and injuries of the head; and diseases of the brain, including epilepsy, various kinds of headache, tinnitus, vertigo, amnesia, and nightmare.

Discourse 3 (12 chapters) on diseases of the eyes and eyelids, the ear and the nose (including epistaxis and catarrh), the face, mouth and teeth.

Discourse 4 (7 chapters) on nervous diseases, including spasm, tetanus, paralysis, facial palsy, etc.

Discourse 5 (7 chapters) on diseases of the throat, chest and vocal organs, including asthma.

Discourse 6 (6 chapters) on diseases of the stomach, including hiccough.

Discourse 7 (5 chapters) on diseases of the liver, including dropsy.

Discourse 8 (14 chapters) on diseases of the heart, lungs, gall-bladder and spleen.

Discourse 9 (19 chapters) on diseases of the intestines (especially colic), and of the urinary and genital organs.

Discourse 10 (26 chapters) on fevers, ephemeral, hectic, continuous, tertian, quartan and semi-quartan; on pleurisy, erysipelas, and small-pox; on crises, prognosis, favourable and unfavourable symptoms, and the signs of death.

Discourse 11 (13 chapters) on rheumatism, gout, sciatica, leprosy, elephantiasis, scrofula, lupus, cancer, tumours, gangrene, wounds and bruises, shock, and plague. The last four chapters deal with anatomical matters, including the numbers of the muscles, nerves and blood-vessels.

Discourse 12 (20 chapters) on phlebotomy, cupping, baths and the indications afforded by the pulse and urine.

This Fourth Part constitutes nearly two-fifths of the whole book, occupying 107 out of 276 folios and comprising in all 152 chapters. Each chapter is therefore very short, often less than one page and seldom more than two. There is little attempt to go beyond the chief signs and symptoms of each disease and the treatment recommended, and, so far as I have seen, there are no references to actual cases, or clinical notes. The book, indeed, except for the First Part—which deals with general philosophic conceptions, and contains some interesting ideas regarding the genesis of the Four Elements (Earth, Air, Fire and Water) from the Four Natures (Heat, Cold, Dryness and Moisture) and their metamorphosis (الاستحالة)—is little more than a Practitioner's Vade-mecum, chiefly interesting as one of the earliest extant independent medical works in Arabic written by the teacher of the great physician whom we have now to consider.

Abú Bakr Muḥammad ibn Zakariyyá of Ray, hence called in Arabic ar-Rází, and by the medieval Latinists "Rhazes," was probably the greatest and most original of all the Muslim physicians, and one of the most prolific as an author. His birth-place, Ray, situated a few miles from Ṭihrán, the modern capital of Persia, was one of the most ancient Persian cities, being mentioned in the *Avesta*[1] as "Ragha of the three races," the twelfth of the good lands created by Ahura Mazda. In early life music was his chief interest, and he was a skilful player on the lute. He then devoted himself to Philosophy, but, according to the Qáḍí Ṣá'id[2], "did not fathom Metaphysics, nor apprehend its ultimate aim, so that his judgment was troubled and he adopted indefensible views, espoused objectionable [*i.e.* heterodox] doctrines, and criticized people whom he did not understand, and whose methods he did not follow." Herein he stands in sharp contrast with Avicenna, of whom we shall speak

---

[1] *Vendîdâd*, Fargard ii, v. 16.
[2] Ibn Abí Uṣaybi'a, i, p. 310.

presently; for Avicenna was a better philosopher than physician, but Rází a better physician than philosopher. Rází, as Ibn Abí Uṣaybi'a informs us, spent most of his life in Persia, because it was his native country, and because his brother and his kinsmen dwelt there. His interest in Medicine was aroused, when he was of mature age, by visits to the hospital and conversations with an old druggist or dispenser who served in it. Of the hospital at Ray he ultimately became chief physician, and there he attended regularly, surrounded by his pupils and the pupils of his pupils. Every patient who presented himself was first examined by the latter—the clinical clerks, as we should say; and if the case proved too difficult for them it was passed on to the Master's immediate pupils, and finally, if necessary, to himself. Subsequently Rází became physician-in-chief to the great hospital at Baghdád, about the foundation of which he is said to have been consulted. Being asked to select the most suitable site, he is said to have caused pieces of meat to be hung up in different quarters of the city, and to have chosen the place where they were slowest in showing signs of decomposition. While in Persia he enjoyed the friendship and patronage of Manṣúr ibn Isḥáq, the ruler of Khurásán, for whom he composed his *Kitábu'l-Manṣúrí* (the "Liber Al-mansoris"). The chronology of his life is very uncertain, for not only do the dates assigned to his death vary between A.D. 903 and 923[1] but he has even been associated by some writers[2] with the great Buwayhid

---

[1] Ibn Abí Uṣaybi'a, i, p. 314.

[2] *Ibid.*, pp. 309–310, but the author expresses the correct opinion that Rází was antecedent to 'Aḍudu'd-Dawla, and that the hospital with which he was connected only received the name of *'Aḍudí* at a later date.

ruler 'Adudu'd-Dawla, who reigned from A.D. 949–982, and who founded the *Bímáristánu'l-'Adudí*, or 'Adudí Hospital, the site of which Rází is said to have selected as described above, at the end of his reign.

One detail occurring in all the accounts of Rází is that he became blind towards the end of his life from a cataract, and that he refused to undergo an operation on the ground that he desired to see no more of a world with which he was disgusted and disillusioned. The indirect cause of his blindness is further stated to have been his preoccupation with Alchemy, on which, as we know from the list of his writings given by al-Qiftí and Ibn Abí Usaybi'a, he composed twelve treatises. One of them he dedicated and presented to a certain great man, who gave him a large reward, and then bade him apply his science to the actual production of gold. Rází made various excuses for declining this test, whereupon the great man lost his temper, accused him of fraud and charlatanism, and struck him a blow on the head which caused him to go blind. Other writers assert that he was secretly strangled for his failure, while others ascribe his blindness to the excessive eating of beans, of which he was very fond. In short his biographers have sought to compensate us for the meagre and conflicting details of his career which they offer us by just such extraordinary stories as gathered round the natural philosophers of the Middle Ages in Europe, where every student of science who transcended his age was suspected of being a magician.

When we turn to the writings of Rází, however, we are on surer ground, for there is no reason to doubt the accuracy of the list of those given by the three most trustworthy biographers, and said to be based on the author's own notes and statements. The *Fihrist*, our oldest authority, enumerates 113 major and 28 minor works by him, besides two poems. Most of these are lost, but what remain are amply sufficient to enable us to appraise his learning, though even of these but few are accessible save in manuscript. Of his many monographs the most celebrated in Europe is his well-known treatise on small-pox and measles, first published in the original Arabic with a Latin translation by Channing (London, 1766). Of this a Latin translation had already appeared in Venice in 1565, and an English version by Greenhill was published by the Sydenham Society in 1848. This tract was formerly known as *de Peste* or *de Pestilentiâ*, and, as Neuburger says[1], "on every hand and with justice it is regarded as an ornament to the medical literature of the Arabs." "It ranks high in importance," he continues, "in the history of epidemiology as the earliest monograph upon small-pox, and shows us Rhazes as a conscientious practitioner, almost free from dogmatic prejudices, following in the footsteps of Hippocrates."

Another monograph by Rází on stone in the bladder and kidneys has been published in the original, with a French translation (Leyden, 1896), by Dr P. de Koning, who has also published the text and translation of the anatomical portion of the *Kitábu'l-Hâwí*, or "Continens," together with the corresponding portions of the *Kitábu'l-Malikí*, or "Liber Regius," of 'Alí ibnu'l-'Abbás and the *Qánún* of Avicenna. To Steinschneider we are indebted for German translations of other tracts by Rází, notably his entertaining work on the success of charlatans and quacks in securing a popularity often denied to the competent and properly qualified physician[2].

---

[1] Ernest Playfair's translation, vol. i, p. 362.
[2] Virchow's *Archiv*, vol. xxxvi, pp. 570–586.

Other unpublished monographs by Rází exist in various public libraries in Europe and the East. Thus a MS. (**Add.** 3516) recently acquired by purchase by the Cambridge University Library contains the treatises on gout and rheumatism[1] and on colic[2] mentioned by al-Qiftí. Of general works on Medicine, apart from his numerous monographs, Rází composed some half dozen, to wit the *Jámi'* or "Compendium," the *Káfí* or "Sufficient," the Lesser and the Greater *Madkhal* or "Introduction," the *Mulúkí* or "Royal," compiled for 'Alí ibn Veh-Súdhán the ruler of Tabaristán, the *Fákhir* or "Splendid" (of which, however, the authorship seems to be uncertain), and last but not least the *Mansúrí* or "Liber Almansoris," of which a Latin translation was published in A.D. 1489, and the *Háwí* or "Continens," of which a Latin translation was published in A.D. 1486 at Brescia, and again at Venice in A.D. 1542. This translation is very rare, and the only copy at Cambridge is in the Library of King's College[3]. It is of the *Háwí* or "Continens" only that I propose to speak, since it is by far the largest and most important of Rází's works.

Unfortunately the study of the *Háwí* is fraught with peculiar difficulties. Not only has it never been published in the original, but no complete manuscript exists, and, indeed, so far as my present knowledge goes, I doubt if more than half of this immense work exists at all at the present day, while the extant volumes are widely dispersed, three volumes in the British Museum, three in the Bodleian, four or five in the Escorial, others at Munich and Petrograd and some abridgments in

---

[1] Ff. 110–142.   [2] Ff. 48–62.
[3] Its class-mark is **xv. 4. 2.**

Berlin. Moreover there is some uncertainty as to the number and contents of the volumes which the work comprises, for while the *Fihrist*[1] enumerates only 12, the Latin translation contains 25, nor is there any correspondence in subject-matter or arrangement. This confusion arises partly, no doubt, from the fact that the *Ḥáwí* was a posthumous work, compiled after the death of Rází by his pupils from unfinished notes and papers which he left behind him, and lacking the unity of plan and finishing touches which only the author's hand could give, and partly from the fact that the same title seems to have been sometimes applied to another of his larger works. Moreover the *Ḥáwí*, on account of its enormous size and the mass of detail which it contained, appalled the most industrious copyists, and was beyond the reach of all save the most wealthy bibliophiles, so that 'Alí ibnu'l-'Abbás, of whom I shall next speak, and who wrote only 50 or 60 years after Rází's death, tells us that in his day he only knew of two complete copies[2]. From what original the Latin translation was made, and whether or where that original now exists, we are unfortunately ignorant, since the medieval translators did not condescend to mention such details. In face of these difficulties all that I have been able to do is to examine superficially the half dozen volumes in the British Museum and the Bodleian Libraries. Of these the most interesting is **Marsh 156** of the latter library, and in particular ff. 239 *b*–245 *b*, of which, through the kindness of Dr Cowley and Professor Margoliouth, I have obtained photographs.

I have already said, and indeed it has been generally

---

[1] p. 300.

[2] *Kámilu'ṣ-Ṣiná'at* (=*al-Kitábu'l-Malikí*), Cairo edition of 1294/1877, vol. i, pp. 5–6.

recognized by all authorities on this subject, that it is
as a clinical observer that Rází excels all his compeers;
and since the clinical notes of these old "Arabian"
physicians are of much greater interest and importance
than their obsolete physiology and pathology or their
second-hand anatomy, a careful study of the works of
Rází, especially of his great *Háwí* or "Continens," is
probably the most repaying field to which the Arabic
scholar interested in Medicine can devote himself.
Some of his more celebrated and sensational cases are
recorded in such collections of anecdotes as the Arabic
Kitábu'l-Faraj ba'da 'sh-Shidda ("Book of Relief after
Distress") of at-Tanúkhí (d. A.D. 994), and the Persian
Chahár Maqála ("Four Discourses"), compiled by
Niẓámí-i-'Arúḍí of Samarqand about A.D. 1155. Ibn
Abí Uṣaybi'a says in his *Classes of Physicians*[1], "There
are many accounts and various valuable observations by ar-Rází as to what he achieved by his skill
in the Art of Medicine, his unique attainments in the
healing of the sick, his deduction of their condition
through his skill in prognosis, and the information which
he gave as to their symptoms and treatment, unto the
like of which but few physicians have attained. He has
many narratives of what fell within his experience in
these and like matters, which are contained in many of
his works."

Now the dozen pages in the Bodleian MS. referred
to above (supposed to be the seventh volume of the
Háwí, but agreeing better with the seventeenth of the
Latin translation[2]), contain precisely such clinical notes
as are mentioned by Ibn Abí Uṣaybi'a. They are

---

[1] Vol. i, p. 311.

[2] Book vii of the Latin translation is entitled *De passionibus cordis
et epatis et splenis*; Book xvii *De effimerâ et ethicâ* (? *hecticâ*).

entitled "Illustrative accounts of patients, and narratives of unusual cases about which we were doubtful[1]."
Some twenty-four cases are recorded, the full names of
the patients being usually given, with the symptoms,
treatment and results. They are not easy to understand,
the Arabic text being represented by one manuscript
only, and the style, apart from apparent scribe's errors,
being crabbed and technical. The first case, which I
interpret as well as I can, may serve as a specimen.

كان يأتى عبد الله بن سواده حمّيات مخلّطة تنوب مرّةً فى ستّة
ايّام و مرّةً غب و مرّةً ربع و مرّةً كلّ يوم و يتقدّمها نافضٌ يسيرٌ و
كان يبول مرّات كثيرة و حكمْتُ انّه لا يخلو أن تكون هذه الحمّيات
تُريد أن تنقلب ربعًا و امّا أن يكون به خراجٌ فى كلاهُ فلم يلبث
الّا مديدة حتّى بال مدّةً أَعْلَمْتُهُ انّه لا يعاود هذه الحمّيات و كان
كذلك و انّما صدّنى فى اوّل الأمر عن أن ابتّ القول بأن به خراجاً
فى كلاهُ انّه كان يحمّر قبل ذلك حمّى غب و حمّيات أُخَر فكان
للظنّ بأن تلك الحمّى المخلّطة من احتراقات تُريد أن تصير ربعًا
موضعًا اقوى و لمريشكُ الىّ أَنْ قَطَنَهُ شبه ثقل معلّق منه اذا قامر و
أغفلْتُ أنا ايضًا أن أسأله عنه و قد كان كثرة البول يقوّى ظنّى
بالخراج فى الكُلى الّا أتى كُنْتُ لا أعلمُ[2] أن أباه ايضًا ضعيف
المثانة يعتريه هذا الدّاء و هو ايضًا قد كان يعتريه فى صحّته
فينبغى أن لا يفعل بعد ذلك غاية التقصّى ان شاء الله، و لمّا بال
المدّة اكببْتُ عليه بما يُدرّ البول حتّى صفا البولُ من المدّة ثمّ سقيْتُهُ
بعد ذلك الطين المختوم و الكندر و دمر الأخوَيْن و تخلص من علّته
و برأ بروًا تامًّا سريعًا فى نَحْوٍ من شهرَيْنِ و كان الخراج صغيرًا و

دلّتى على ذلك انّه لم يشك الىّ ابتداءً ثقلاً فى قَطَنِه لكن بعد أن
بال مِدَّةً قلْتُ له هل كنْتَ تجد ذلك قال نعم فلو كان كثيرًا لقد
كان يشكو ذلك وان المِدَّة تُنْبَثُ سريعًا تدلّ على صغر الخراج فأمّا
غيرى من الاطبّاء فأتّهم كانوا بعد أن بال مِدَّةً ايضًا لا يعلمون حالته
البتّةَ ،

"'Abdu'lláh ibn Sawáda used to suffer from attacks of mixed fever, sometimes quotidian, sometimes tertian, sometimes quartan, and sometimes recurring once in six days. These attacks were preceded by a slight rigor, and micturition was very frequent. I gave it as my opinion that either these accesses of fever would turn into quartan, or that there was ulceration of the kidneys. Only a short while elapsed ere the patient passed pus in his urine. I thereupon informed him that these feverish attacks would not recur, and so it was.

"The only thing which prevented me at first from giving it as my definite opinion that the patient was suffering from ulceration of the kidneys was that he had previously.suffered from tertian and other mixed types of fever, and this to some extent confirmed my suspicion that this mixed fever might be from inflammatory processes which would tend to become quartan when they waxed stronger.

"Moreover the patient did not complain to me that his loins felt like a weight depending from him when he stood up; and I neglected to ask him about this. The frequent micturition also should have strengthened my suspicion of ulceration of the kidneys, but I did not know that his father suffered from weakness of the bladder and was subject to this complaint, and it used likewise to come upon him when he was healthy[1], and it ought not to be the case henceforth, till the end of his life, if God will.

"So when he passed the pus I administered to him diuretics until the urine became free from pus, after which I treated him with *terra sigillata*, Boswellia thurifera, and Dragon's Blood, and his sickness departed from him, and he was quickly and completely cured in about two months. That the ulceration was slight was indicated to me by the fact that he did not complain to me at first of weight in the loins. After he had passed pus, however, I enquired of him whether he had experienced this symptom, and he replied in the affirmative. Had the

---

[1] *I.e.* before he suffered from fever.

ulceration been extensive, he would of his own accord have complained of this symptom. And that the pus was evacuated quickly indicated a limited ulceration. The other physicians whom he consulted besides myself, however, did not understand the case at all, even after the patient had passed pus in his urine."

In spite of several difficulties, both verbal and material, which I have not yet been able to solve to my satisfaction, the general nature of this case seems fairly clear. The patient suffered from intermittent and irregular attacks of fever preceded by slight rigors, which, in a land infested with ague, were diagnosed and treated as malarial, though really septic in origin. Rází himself at first took this view, but subsequently, observing the presence of pus in the urine, diagnosed the case as one of pyelitis, and treated it accordingly with success.

We now come to the third name in our list, 'Alí ibnu'l-'Abbás, known in Europe in the Middle Ages as "Haly Abbas," of whose *Kitábu'l-Malikí*, or "Liber Regius," the Latin translation by "Stephen the Philosopher," with annotations by Michael de Capella, was printed at Lyons in 1523. The notice of him given by al-Qiftí[1] is so short that it may be translated in full :

"Alí ibnu'l-'Abbás al-Majúsí (the Magian or Zoroastrian), an accomplished and perfect physician of Persian origin, known as 'the son of the Magian.' He studied with a Persian professor (*Shaykh*) known as Abú Máhir [Músá ibn Sayyár], and also studied and worked by himself, and acquainted himself with the writings of the ancients. He composed for the King 'Adudu'd-Dawla Fanákhusraw the Buwayhid[2] his System of Medicine entitled *al-Malikí* ("the Royal"), which is a splendid work and a noble thesaurus comprehending the science and practice of Medicine, admirably arranged.

[1] p. 232.   [2] Reigned 949–982.

It enjoyed great popularity in its day and was diligently studied, until the appearance of Avicenna's *Qánún*, which usurped its popularity and caused the *Malikí* to be somewhat neglected. The latter excels on the practical and the former on the scientific side."

The *Fihrist* no longer serves us, as it was completed at a date antecedent to that of which we are now speaking, and the only important particular added by Ibn Abí Uṣaybi'a[1] is that 'Alí ibnu'l-'Abbás was a native of Ahwáz in S.W. Persia, not far from the once great medical school of Jundí-Shápúr of which so much was said in the last lecture ; while his *nisba* or title of al-Majúsí indicates that his father or grandfather originally belonged to the old Persian religion of Zoroaster. Neither he nor his master Abú Máhir wrote much; the *Malikí* is the only work ascribed to him by the biographers, though Brockelmann[2] mentions a MS. at Gotha containing another medical treatise attributed to him, while only two works by his master are mentioned, a treatise on phlebotomy, and a supplement to one of Isḥáq ibn Ḥunayn's smaller manuals on practical Medicine.

Although we know no more of the life of 'Alí ibnu 'l-'Abbás than the meagre details just mentioned, and of his date only that he was contemporary with the great and enlightened 'Aḍudu'd-Dawla, the founder of the 'Aḍudí Hospital at Baghdád, who flourished in the latter half of the tenth century, his work, the *Malikí* or "Liber Regius," is the most accessible and most readable of the great Arabic Systems of Medicine, since an excellent edition in two volumes was printed at Cairo in 1294/1877, and the Latin version, though rare, is

---

[1] Vol. i, pp. 236–7.
[2] *Gesch. d. Arab. Litt.*, vol. i, p. 237.

fortunately not included amongst the *Incunabula*, and can therefore be borrowed from the libraries which possess it. The Arabic text comprises some 400,000 words, and is divided into 20 Discourses, each subdivided into numerous chapters, of which the first ten deal with the theory, and the second ten with the practice of Medicine. The second and third of these Discourses, dealing with Anatomy, have been published with a French translation by Dr P. de Koning (Leyden, 1903) in his *Trois Traités d'Anatomie Arabes* (pp. 90–431). The nineteenth Discourse, containing 110 chapters, is devoted entirely to Surgery[1].

The introductory portion of the book, comprising the first three chapters of the first Discourse, is very well written and very interesting, especially the criticism of previous works on Medicine. Of the Greek physicians he discusses especially Hippocrates, Galen, Oribasius and Paul of Ægina; of the Syrians and Muslims, Ahrún the Priest, Yuḥanná ibn Serapion, and ar-Rází. He finds Hippocrates too concise and hence sometimes obscure, and Galen too diffuse; he criticizes Oribasius and Paul of Ægina for omitting or dealing inadequately with Anatomy, Surgery, Natural Philosophy, Humoral Pathology, and the Ætiology of disease. Of the moderns he finds the work of Ahrún alone adequate in its scope, but complains of the badness and obscurity of the Arabic translation. Ibn Serapion, he says, ignores Surgery, omits all mention of many important diseases which he enumerates, including Aneurism, and arranges his materials badly and unsystematically. I have already alluded to his observations on the enormous size and prolixity of Rází's "Continens," which placed it beyond the reach of all save the very wealthy, and so led to an

---

[1] pp. 454–516 of vol. ii of the Cairo edition.

extreme scarcity of manuscripts, even within a short time of the author's death, while Rází's other and better-known work the *Mansúrí* he finds unduly concise. He then explains the plan of his own book, in which he seeks to find a *via media* between undue conciseness and prolixity, and illustrates his method by a specimen description of pleurisy. He begins with the definition of the disease and its aetiology ; then proceeds to the four constant symptoms, fever, cough, pain and dyspnoea; whence he passes to the prognosis, and especially the indications furnished by the sputa, and concludes with the treatment. His remarks at the end of this chapter on the importance of regular attendance at the hospitals are worth quoting[1].

"And of those things which are incumbent on the student of this Art are that he should constantly attend the hospitals and sick-houses; pay unremitting attention to the conditions and circumstances of their inmates, in company with the most acute professors of Medicine; and enquire frequently as to the state of the patients and the symptoms apparent in them, bearing in mind what he has read about these variations, and what they indicate of good or evil. If he does this, he will reach a high degree in this Art. Therefore it behoves him who desires to be an accomplished physician to follow closely these injunctions, to form his character in accordance with what we have mentioned therein, and not to neglect them. If he does this, his treatment of the sick will be successful ; people will have confidence in him and be favourably disposed towards him, and he will win their affection and respect and a good reputa-

[1] Vol. i, p. 9. The corresponding passage in the Latin translation occurs in the upper part of the left-hand column of f. 7 *b* of the Lyons edition of A.D. 1523.

tion; nor withal will he lack profit and advantage from them. And God Most High knoweth best."

In connection with the concluding words of the above extract, something may be said here as to the fees earned by one of the most eminent physicians under the early 'Abbásid Caliphs, viz. Jibrá'íl ibn Bukht-Yishú', who died about A.D. 830. According to al-Qiftí[1] he received out of the public funds a monthly salary of 10,000 *dirhams*, and from the Privy Purse 50,000 *dirhams* at the beginning of each year, besides clothes to the value of 10,000 *dirhams*. For bleeding the Caliph Hárúnu'r-Rashíd twice a year he was paid 100,000 *dirhams*, and an equal sum for administering a biennial purgative draught. From the nobles of the Court he received in cash and kind 400,000 *dirhams* a year, and from the great Barmecide family 1,400,000 *dirhams*. According to al-Qiftí's computation, the total amount which he received in these ways, apart from what he earned privately from lesser patients, during his 23 years' service of Hárúnu'r-Rashíd and his 13 years' service of the Barmecides, amounted to 88,800,000 *dirhams*, a sum equivalent, if we accept von Kremer's[2] estimate of the *dirham* as roughly equivalent to a franc, to more than three and a half million pounds sterling.

I come now to the last and most famous of the four Persian physicians of whom I propose to speak to-day, viz. Avicenna, or, to give him his correct name, Abú 'Alí Husayn ibn 'Abdu'lláh ibn Síná, generally entitled *ash-Shaykhu'r-Ra'ís*, the "Chief Master," or *al-Mu 'allimu'th-Thání*, the "Second Teacher," to wit after Aristotle. The difficulty here is to decide what to say

[1] pp. 142–3.
[2] *Culturgeschichte d. Orients*, vol. i, p. 15 *ad calc.*

out of so much that deserves mention, for in Avicenna,
philosopher, physician, poet and man of affairs, the so-
called Arabian science culminates, and is, as it were,
personified. In the limits prescribed to me it would be
impossible to enumerate his multitudinous writings on
philosophy and science, or to narrate the details of a
life of which he himself kept a record, still preserved
to us, up to his twenty-first year, and of which the
remainder has been recorded by his pupil and friend
Abú 'Ubayd of Júzján. His father, an adherent of the
Isma'ílí sect, was from Balkh and his mother from a
village near Bukhárá, and he was born about A.D. 980.
At the age of ten he was already proficient in the
Qur'án and the Arabic classics. During the six succeeding years he devoted himself to Muslim Jurisprudence,
Philosophy and Natural Science, and studied Logic,
Euclid, the 'Εισαγωγή, and the *Almagest*. He turned
his attention to Medicine at the age of sixteen, and
found it "not difficult," but was greatly troubled by
metaphysical problems, until, by a fortunate chance, he
obtained possession of a small and cheap manual by
the celebrated philosopher al-Fárábí, which solved his
difficulties. When he was not much more than eighteen
years old his reputation as a physician was such that he
was summoned to attend the Sámání ruler Núh ibn
Mansúr (reigned A.D. 976–997), who, in gratitude for
his services, allowed him to make free use of the royal
library, which contained many rare and even unique
books. This library was subsequently destroyed by fire,
and Avicenna's detractors did not scruple to assert that
he himself had purposely burned it so as to enjoy a
monopoly of the learning he had derived from it. At
the age of twenty-one he lost his father, and about the
same time composed his first book. He entered the

service of 'Alí ibn Ma'mún, the ruler of Khwárazm or Khiva, for a while, but ultimately fled thence to avoid the attempt of Sulṭán Mahmúd of Ghazna to kidnap him. After many wanderings he came to Jurján, attracted by the fame of its ruler Qábús as a patron of learning, but the deposition and murder of that prince almost coincided with his arrival, and he bitterly exclaimed in a poem which he composed on this occasion:

لّما عظمْتُ فليس مصرٌ واسعى، لّما غلا ثمنى عدمْتُ المشترى،

"*When I became great no country had room for me;
When my price went up I lacked a purchaser.*"

Such a "purchaser," however, he ultimately found in the Amír Shamsu'd-Dawla of Hamadán, whom he cured of the colic, and who made him his Prime Minister. A mutiny of the soldiers against him caused his dismissal and imprisonment, but subsequently the Amír, being again attacked by the colic, summoned him back, apologized to him, and reinstated him. His life at this time was extraordinarily strenuous; all day he was busy with the Amír's service, while a great part of the night was passed in lecturing and dictating notes for his books, with intervals of wine-drinking and minstrelsy. After many vicissitudes, which time forbids me to enumerate, but which are minutely chronicled by his faithful friend and disciple Abú 'Ubayd of Júzján, Avicenna, worn out by hard work and hard living, died in 428/1036–7 at the comparatively early age of 58. In his last illness he treated himself unsuccessfully, so that it was said by his detractors that neither could his physic save his body nor his metaphysics his soul[1].

[1] The verses in question are given by Ibn Abí Uṣaybi'a (*Ṭaba-qátu'l-Aṭibbá*, vol. ii, p. 6), and in the notes to my forthcoming translation of the *Chahár Maqála* ("E. J. W. Gibb Memorial" Series, vol. xi, 2, p. 156).

His writings were numerous and in many cases voluminous, some of his major works comprising as many as twenty volumes. The professedly complete list of them given by al-Qifṭí[1] includes the titles of 21 major and 24 minor works on philosophy, medicine, theology, geometry, astronomy, philology and the like. Most of these are in Arabic; but in Persian, his native language, he wrote one large book, a manual of philosophical sciences entitled *Dánish-náma-i-'Alá'í* (represented by a MS. in the British Museum[2]), and a small treatise on the Pulse. The list given by Brockelmann in his *Geschichte der Arabischen Litteratur* (vol. i, pp. 452–458), which includes only extant works, is, however, much more extensive than al-Qifṭí's, and comprises 68 books on theology and metaphysics, 11 on astronomy and natural philosophy, 16 on medicine, and 4 in verse, 99 books in all. His most celebrated Arabic poem is that describing the descent of the Soul into the Body from the Higher Sphere (الأرفع المحلّ) which is its home, a poem of real beauty, of which a translation is given in my *Literary History of Persia* (vol. ii, pp. 110–111). The industry of the late Dr Ethé has also collected from various biographical works 15 short Persian poems, mostly quatrains, comprising in all some forty verses, which are ascribed to Avicenna. Of these the best known is commonly, but probably falsely, ascribed to 'Umar Khayyám, at least one fifth of whose reputed quatrains are attributed on as good or better evidence to other people. The quatrain in question is the one translated by FitzGerald:

[1] Ed. Lippert, p. 418.

[2] **Or. 16, 830.** See Rieu's *Pers. Cat.*, pp. 433–4. Mr A. G. Ellis has called my attention to a lithographed edition of this work, published in India in 1309/1891.

"*Up from Earth's Centre through the Seventh Gate
I rose, and on the Throne of Saturn sate,
And many a knot unravelled by the Road,
But not the Master-knot of Human Fate.*"

The original, as given in the *Majma'u'l-Fuṣaḥá*[1], runs
as follows:

از قعر ِ گِلِ سیاه تا اوج زحل ، کردم همه مشکلاتِ گیتی را حلّ ،

بیرون جَستم زقیدِ هر مکر و حیل ، هر بند گشاده شد مگر بندِ اجل ،

Of Avicenna's medical works exactly half, viz. 8, are
versified treatises on such matters as the 25 signs indicating the fatal termination of illnesses, hygienic precepts, proved remedies, anatomical memoranda, and the
like. One or two of them have been published in the
East, but I have not seen them. I imagine, however,
that they are of little value either as verse or as science.
Of his prose works, after the great *Qánún*, the treatise
on Cardiac Drugs (الأدوية القلبيّة), of which the British
Museum possesses several fine old manuscripts, is
probably the most important, but it remains unpublished,
and is inaccessible beyond the walls of that and a few
other great public libraries[2].

The *Qánún* is, of course, by far the largest, the
most famous, and the most important of Avicenna's
medical works, and at the same time the most accessible,
both in the original Arabic and in the Latin translation
of Gerard of Cremona. There is a modern Egyptian
edition of the Arabic text, besides the Roman edition of
A.D. 1593; and a fine Venetian translation into Latin
published in 1544. The work contains not much less
than a million words, and, like most Arabic books, is

---

[1] Vol. i, p. 68.
[2] Berlin, Gotha, Leyden, and the Escorial.

elaborately divided and subdivided. The main division is into five Books, of which the first treats of general principles; the second of simple drugs arranged alphabetically; the third of diseases of particular organs and members of the body, from the head to the feet; the fourth of diseases which, though local and partial in their inception, tend to spread to other parts of the body, such as fevers; and the fifth of compound medicines. These descriptions are in fact very inadequate. Thus Book IV treats not only of fevers, but of critical days, prognosis, tumours and ulcers, fractures, dislocations and toxicology.

I had intended to discuss this great and celebrated book more fully than the time at my disposal to-day actually allows, but this is of the less consequence inasmuch as the College has done me the honour of inviting me to deliver the FitzPatrick lectures again next year, when I hope to recur to it in connection with the topics of which I shall then have to treat. Its encyclopaedic character, its systematic arrangement, its philosophic plan, perhaps even its dogmatism, combined with the immense reputation of its author in other fields besides Medicine, raised it to a unique position in the medical literature of the Muslim world, so that the earlier works of ar-Rází and al-Majúsí, in spite of their undoubted merits, were practically abrogated by it, and it is still regarded in the East by the followers of the old Greek Medicine, the *Tibb-i-Yúnání*, as the last appeal on all matters connected with the healing art. In proof of this statement, and to show the extraordinary reverence in which Avicenna is held, I will conclude with a quotation from that pleasant work the *Chahár Maqála*, or "Four Discourses," composed in Persian in the middle of the twelfth century of our era, and dealing with four classes

of men, to wit Secretaries of State, Poets, Astrologers
and Physicians, deemed by the author, Niẓámí-i-'Arúḍí
of Samarqand, indispensable for the service of kings.
After enumerating a number of books which should be
diligently studied by him who aspires to eminence in
Medicine, the author says that if he desires to be independent of all other works he may rest satisfied with
the *Qánún*, and thus continues[1]:

"The Lord of the two Worlds and Guide of the
two Material Races saith: '*Every kind of game is com-
prehended in the Wild Ass.*' All this, together with
much more, is to be found in the *Qánún*, and from him
who hath mastered the first volume thereof nothing
will be hidden concerning the general theory and
principles of Medicine, so that could Hippocrates and
Galen return to life, it would be proper that they should
do reverence to this book. Yet have I heard a wonderful
thing, to wit that one hath taken exception to Abú 'Alí
[Avicenna] in respect to this work, and hath embodied
his criticisms in a book which he hath entitled the
Rectification of the Qánún. It is as though I looked
upon both, and saw how foolish is the author and how
detestable his work. For what right hath anyone to find
fault with so great a man, when the very first question
he meets with in a book of his which he comes across
is difficult to his comprehension? For four thousand
years the physicians of antiquity travailed in spirit and
spent their very souls in order to reduce the science of

[1] The passage cited occurs on pp. 70-71 of the text of the *Chahár
Maqála* published in 1910 in the "E. J. W. Gibb Memorial" Series,
vol. xi, and on pp. 110-111 of the separate reprint of the translation
which I published in 1899 in the *Journal of the Royal Asiatic Society.*
In my new revised translation, which will appear shortly as vol. xi, 2
of the Gibb Series, it will be found on pp. 79-80.

Philosophy to some fixed order, yet could they not effect this; until after the lapse of this period that pure philosopher and most great thinker Aristotle weighed out this coin in the balance of Logic, assayed it with the touchstone of Definitions, and measured it with the measure of Analogy, so that all doubt and uncertainty departed from it, and it was established on a sure and critical basis. And during these fifteen centuries which have elapsed since his time, no philosopher has won to the inmost essence of his doctrine, nor travelled the high road of his pre-eminence save that most excellent of the moderns, the Philosopher of the East, the Proof of God to mankind, Abú 'Alí Husayn ibn 'Abdu'lláh ibn Síná [Avicenna]. Whosoever, therefore, finds fault with these two great men will have cast himself out from the fellowship of the wise, ranked himself with madmen, and revealed himself as fit company only for fools. May God by His Grace and Favour keep us from such stumblings and vain imaginings!"

LECTURE III

Before proceeding further with my subject, it may, perhaps, be well that I should recapitulate very briefly the main points I endeavoured to establish in the two lectures which I had the honour of delivering before you last year. I pointed out that the term "Arabian Medicine" (to which "Islamic Medicine" would be preferable) can be justified only if we regard the language which serves as its vehicle, and the auspices under which it was evolved; that it was an eclectic synthesis of more ancient systems, chiefly Greek, but in a lesser degree Indian and old Persian, with a tincture of other exotic systems less easily to be identified; and that the Medicine of the Arabian people at the time of their Prophet's advent, that is in the early seventh century of the Christian era, was, as it continues to be, of the most primitive type. In this connection I referred to the observations of Dr Zwemer in his *Arabia, the Cradle of Islâm*, and I must now add a reference to a very interesting little book in Arabic by an Egyptian doctor, 'Abdu'r-Raḥmán Efendi Isma'íl, published at Cairo in 1892 or 1893, on the popular medicine and medical superstitions of his countrymen, and, still more, of his countrywomen. This system, if such it can be called, is entitled *Ṭibbu'r-Rukka*[1], roughly equivalent in meaning to "Old Wives' Medicine," and is fiercely exposed and denounced by the author, who regards its survival until

---

[1] On the word *Rukka*, which is apparently borrowed from the Italian *rocco*, see an interesting observation by Vollers in vol. xxi of the *Z. D. M. G.* (1897), p. 322.

the present day in a country like Egypt, supposed to be in touch with modern enlightenment, as an abomination.

In the development of Arabian Medicine in the wider sense, that is to say, the adaptation of ancient Greek Medicine to the general system of civilization and science eclectically built up by Muslim scholars and thinkers during the "Golden Prime" of the Caliphate of Baghdád, namely from the middle of the eighth century of our era onwards, I distinguished two periods, that of the translation into Arabic of the masterpieces of Greek medical literature, destined to form the basis of further study; and that of the Arabic-speaking or at any rate Arabic-writing physicians (many of whom were Jews, Christians, Sabaeans and even Zoroastrians), who, checking or modifying this material in the light of their own experience, produced more or less independent works. Of these I briefly discussed four of the most notable who flourished in Persia between A.D. 850 and A.D. 1036, the year in which died Abú 'Alí ibn Síná, familiar to the West as Avicenna, the three others being 'Alí ibn Rabban, who composed his "Paradise of Wisdom" for the Caliph al-Mutawakkil in A.D. 850; Abú Bakr Muḥammad ibn Zakariyyá ar-Rází, familiar to medieval Europe as Rhazes; and 'Alí ibnu'l-'Abbás al-Majúsí, called by the Latino-Barbari of the Middle Ages "Haly Abbas." I briefly described four of the chief works of these four great physicians, namely the "Paradise of Wisdom" (which, from its extreme rarity, has hitherto remained unnoticed outside the Arabic Catalogues of the British Museum and Berlin); the *Ḥáwí* or "Continens"; the *Kámilu'ṣ-Ṣiná'at* or "Liber Regius"; and the *Qánún* or "Canon of Medicine" of Avicenna. I further expressed my agreement with the view, advanced by Neuburger, Pagel and other historians of Medicine, that, notwithstanding the greater celebrity achieved by Avicenna, Rází, by virtue of his clinical observations (some of which are preserved to us in a manuscript volume of the *Háwí* in the Bodleian Library[1]), deserves to rank highest of the four, and perhaps of all the physicians produced by Islám during the thirteen centuries of its existence. To his work, and to that of the three other physicians just mentioned, I would gladly recur, should the brief time at my disposal allow, but other matters connected with the history, literature and status of Medicine in the Muslim world demand prior consideration, so that the whole field may be surveyed before any attempt is made to fill in details.

It has been already pointed out that the Muslims were rather the faithful transmitters of the ancient learning of Greece than the creators of a new system. Withington, in his excellent little *Medical History*[2], puts the case so well that I cannot do better than quote his words. " This display of physical vigour," he says, after describing the wonderful conquests of the Arabs in the seventh century, " was followed by an intellectual activity hardly less wonderful. A Byzantine emperor was astonished to find that the right of collecting and purchasing Greek manuscripts was among the terms dictated by a victorious barbarian, and that an illustrated copy of Dioscorides was the most acceptable present he could offer to a friendly chieftain. The philosophers of Constantinople were amazed by the appearance of Muslim writers whom they styled with reluctant admiration 'learned savages,' while the less cultured Christians soon came to look upon the wisdom of the Saracens as something more than human. It was this

---

[1] **Marsh 156**, ff. 239 *b*–246 *a*. See pp. 50–3 *supra*.
[2] The Scientific Press, London, 1894, pp. 138–9.

people who now took from the hands of unworthy successors of Galen and Hippocrates the flickering torch of Greek medicine. They failed to restore its ancient splendour, but they at least prevented its extinction, and they handed it back after five centuries burning more brightly than before."

"Five centuries," however, is an over-statement, for while Avicenna was still in the prime of life there was born in North Africa, probably in Tunis, a man of whose biography little is known, but who was destined to become famous, under the name of Constantinus Africanus, as the first to make known to Western Europe the learning of the Arabs through the medium of the Latin tongue[1]. He attached himself to the celebrated medical school of Salerno—the "Civitas Hippocratica"—and died at Monte Casino, after a life of great literary activity, about A.D. 1087, exactly a century before the still more famous Oriental.scholar and translator Gerard of Cremona. To these two, and to the Jewish physician Faraj ibn Sálim (Fararius or Faragut), who completed his translation of the "Continens" of Rází in A.D. 1279, medieval Europe was chiefly indebted for its knowledge of Arabian Medicine.

The transmission of ideas between East and West was effected, however, through other than literary channels. However great may have been the bitterness of feeling on both sides associated with the Crusades, it is astonishing how much friendly intercourse took place in the intervals of fighting between the Crusaders and their Saracen antagonists. Amongst many somewhat arid chronicles there has been preserved to us, and

---

[1] See an article on his work in vol. xxxvii (pp. 351–410) of Virchow's *Archiv* (Berlin, 1866) by that most erudite Orientalist Moritz Steinschneider.

rendered available by M. Hartwig Derenbourg in the original Arabic accompanied by a French translation[1], the illuminating memoirs of a Saracen Amir named Usáma ibn Munqidh, who flourished in Syria in the twelfth century, and spent most of his life in fighting the Franks. He was born in A.D. 1095, the very year in which the Crusaders captured Antioch and Jerusalem, and died in A.D. 1188. It was during a temporary lull in the fighting between A.D. 1140 and 1143 that his intercourse with the Franks chiefly fell. In his discursive but entertaining memoirs he discusses many of their customs and characteristics which seemed to him curious or enter- taining, and amongst other matters relates several strange stories about their medical practice[2]. At the request of the Frankish Warden of the Castle of Munaytira in the Lebanon, Usáma's uncle sent his Christian physician Thábit to treat certain persons who lay sick there. Ten days later Thábit returned, and was greeted with con- gratulations on the rapidity with which he had cured his patients. For these congratulations, however, there was, as he explained, no occasion. On his arrival they introduced to him two patients, a man suffering from an abscess in the leg, and a consumptive woman. These he proceeded to treat, the first by poultices, the second by suitable diet and drugs. Both were progressing satis- factorily when a Frankish doctor intervened, and, de- nouncing the treatment pursued as useless, turned to the male patient and asked him whether he would prefer to die with two legs or to live with one. The patient expressed his preference for the second alternative, whereupon the Frankish doctor summoned a stalwart

---

[1] Leroux, Paris, 1886–1893.

[2] These will be found on pp. 97–101 of the Arabic text and pp. 491–4 of the French translation.

man-at-arms with an axe, and bade him chop off the patient's leg at one blow. This he failed to do, and at the second blow the marrow was crushed out of the bone and the patient almost immediately expired. The Frankish doctor then turned his attention to the woman, and, after examining her, declared her to be possessed of a devil which was located in her head. He ordered her hair to be shaved off and that she should return to the ordinary diet of her compatriots, garlic and oil; and when she grew worse he made a deep cruciform incision on her head, exposing the bone, and rubbed salt into the wound, whereupon the woman also expired. " After this," concluded Thábit, " I asked if my services were any longer required, and, receiving a negative answer, returned home, having learned of their medical practice what had hitherto been unknown to me."

Usáma relates another similar anecdote on the authority of Guillaume de Bures[1], with whom he travelled from Acre to Tiberias. "There was with us in our country," said Guillaume, "a very doughty knight, who fell ill and was at the point of death. As a last resource we applied to a Christian priest of great authority and entrusted the patient to him, saying, 'Come with us to examine such-and-such a knight.' He agreed and set off with us. Our belief was that he had only to lay hands upon him to cure him. As soon as the priest saw the patient, he said, ' Bring me wax.' We brought him some, and he softened it and made [two plugs] like the joints of a finger, each of which he thrust into one of the patient's nostrils ; whereupon he expired. ' He is dead,' we exclaimed. 'Yes,' replied the priest; ' he was suffering, and I plugged his nostrils so that he might die and be at peace!'"

[1] *Op. cit.*, text, p. 101; translation, p. 494.

To the Arabs of that period, then, as we can well understand, Frankish medicine appeared most barbarous and primitive compared with their own; and it is not surprising that, when Usáma was himself attacked by a chill accompanied by rigors at Shayzar, he preferred the services of an Arab physician, Shaykh Abu'l-Wafá Tamím, to those of a Frankish doctor[1]. Yet, in justice to the Franks, he relates two cases of successful treatment by their medical practitioners; one of a certain Bernard, treasurer to Count Foulques of Anjou, whom Usáma describes as "one of the most accursed of the Franks and the foulest of them," whose death he earnestly desired and prayed for[2]; and the other of the scrofulous child of an Arab artisan named Abu'l-Fath[3]. The former suffered from an injury to the leg caused by a kick from his horse, and fourteen incisions had been made which refused to heal until the Frankish doctor finally consulted removed all the ointments and plasters which had been applied to the wounds, and bathed them with very strong vinegar, as a result of which treatment they gradually healed, and the patient, to quote Usáma's expression, "was cured and arose like the Devil," or, as we should say, ready for any fresh mischief. The scrofulous boy had been taken to Antioch by his father, who had business there, and aroused the compassion of a Frank with whom they foregathered. "Swear to me by thy faith," said he to the father, "that, if I impart to thee a remedy to heal him, thou wilt accept no pecuniary recompense from anyone whom thou mayst treat therewith, and I will give thee the recipe." The father gave the required

---

[1] *Op. cit.*, text, p. 137; translation, p. 491.
[2] *Op. cit.*, text, p. 98; translation, pp. 492–3.
[3] *Op. cit.*, text, pp. 98–9; translation, pp. 493–4.

assurance, and was instructed to take unpounded soda, heat it and mix it with olive oil and strong vinegar, and apply the mixture to the strumous ulcers in the child's neck, this to be followed by the application of what Usáma calls "burnt lead" mixed with butter or grease. The boy, we read, was cured, and the same treatment was subsequently employed with success in other cases.

The above anecdotes do not exhaust the medical material contained in these interesting memoirs. There was a somewhat notable Arab Christian physician named Ibn Butlán who died about A.D. 1063, and was the author of numerous medical works (enumerated by Leclerc[1] and Brockelmann[2]), of the most celebrated of which, the *Taqwímu's-Sihha*, a Latin translation entitled *Tacuini Sanitatis* was printed at Strassburg in A.D. 1531 or 1532. A copy of this work is included amongst the Arabic MSS. of this college. Ibn Butlán, in the course of his extensive travels, was for a time in attendance on Usáma's great-grandfather at Shayzar, and our author records some of the anecdotes about him still current in the household when he was young. One of these is of a dropsical man whose case Ibn Butlán gave up as hopeless, and whom he subsequently met completely cured of his malady. In reply to enquiries as to the treatment which had proved so successful, the man declared no one had attempted to do anything to alleviate his misery except his old mother, who had daily given him a piece of bread soaked in vinegar which she took from a jar. Ibn Butlán asked to see the jar, poured out the remains of the vinegar, and discovered at the bottom two vipers which had fallen into it and become partly macerated or dissolved. " O my

---

[1] *Hist. de la Médecine Arabe*, vol. i, pp. 489–492.

[2] *Gesch. d. Arab. Litt.*, vol. i, p. 483.

son," he exclaimed, "none but God, mighty and glorious is He, could have cured thee with a decoction of vipers in vinegar[1]!"

On another occasion a man came to Ibn Buṭlán in his surgery at Aleppo complaining of hoarseness and complete loss of voice, and stating in reply to enquiries as to his occupation that he was a sifter of earth. Ibn Buṭlán made him drink half a pint of strong vinegar, whereupon he was presently seized with vomiting and threw up a quantity of mud with the vinegar, after which his throat was cleared and his speech became normal. Ibn Buṭlán said to his son and his pupils who were present, "Treat no one with this remedy or you will kill him. As for this man, some of the dust from the sieve had stuck in his gullet and nothing but vinegar could have dislodged it[2]."

I have already observed how general was the interest taken in medical topics in the medieval Muslim world. A very popular branch of literature, both in Arabic and Persian, was constituted by collections of strange and quaint anecdotes, called *Nawádir*, in which the historical or quasi-historical stories are grouped under appropriate headings. In such books a special section is often devoted to Medicine and Physicians. The material thus afforded, though it has not hitherto attracted much attention, appears to me worthy of some notice.

One of the older Arabic books of this sort is a work entitled *al-Faraj ba'da 'sh-Shidda* ("Joy after Sorrow," or better, perhaps, "Relief after Distress") by the Qádí Abu 'Alí at-Tanúkhí, who was born in A.D. 939 and

---

[1] *Op. cit.*, text, p. 135; translation, pp. 488–9.
[2] *Op. cit.*, text, pp. 135–6; translation, p. 489.

died in A.D. 994. This book was printed in Cairo in 1903–4 in two volumes. It comprises 14 chapters, of which the tenth (pp. 94–104 of vol. ii) deals with remarkable cases and contains 15 anecdotes, some of which are trivial or disgusting, while others are of considerable interest. Two of them, which I shall notice first, are connected with the great physician Abú Bakr Muḥammad ibn Zakariyyá ar-Rází (Rhazes) of whom I spoke last year in the second of my two lectures, and with whom our author was almost contemporary.

The first of these[1] is about a young man of Baghdád who came to Rhazes complaining of haematemesis. Careful examination failed to reveal the cause or explain the symptom. The patient was in despair, believing that where Rhazes failed, none could succeed. Rhazes, touched alike by his distress and his faith, then proceeded to question him very carefully as to the water he had drunk on his journey, and ascertained that in some cases it had been drawn from stagnant ponds. "When I come to-morrow," said he to the patient, "I will treat you, and not leave you until you are cured, on condition that you will order your servants to obey me in all that I command them concerning thee." The patient gave the required promise, and Rhazes returned next day with two vessels filled with a water-weed called in Arabic *Ṭuḥlub* and in Persian *Jáma-i-Ghúk* ("Frog's coat") or *Pashm-i-Wazagh*[2] ("Frog's wool"), which he ordered the patient to swallow. The patient, having swallowed a considerable quantity, declared

---

[1] Vol. ii, p. 96. The story is also given by Ibn Abí Uṣaybi'a, vol. i, pp. 311–312.

[2] Identified by Achundow (pp. 231 and 383) with *Lemna* or *Herba Lentis Palustris*, the φακός of Dioscorides, in German *Wasserlinde*. At the present day it is called by the Persians *Jul-i-Wazagh*.

himself unable to take any more, whereupon Rhazes ordered the servants to hold him on his back on the ground and open his mouth, into which he continued to cram more and more of the nauseous substance until violent vomiting ensued. Examination of the vomit revealed a leech which was the source of the trouble, and with the expulsion of which the patient regained his health. This same anecdote occurs in the Persian collection of stories by 'Awfí of which I shall shortly speak, and it is there added that the leech when swallowed in the drinking-water had attached itself to the mouth of the patient's stomach and there remained until induced to transfer itself to the more congenial water-weed.

In the next anecdote[1] Rhazes is represented as describing the case of a dropsical boy whose father consulted him at Bisṭám in N.E. Persia as he was returning from his celebrated cure of the Amír of Khurásán[2], for whom he composed his "Liber Almansoris." Rhazes declared the case to be hopeless, and advised the father to let his son eat and drink whatever he pleased. Twelve months later he returned to the same town, and, to his great astonishment, found the boy completely restored to health. On enquiring how this had come about, he was told that the boy, despairing of health and life, and wishing to put an end to his existence, had one day observed a great snake approach a bowl of *madíra* (a kind of broth prepared with sour milk) which was standing on the ground, drink some of it, and then vomit into the rest, which

---

[1] *Al-Faraj*, vol. ii, pp. 103–104, and Ibn Abí Uṣaybi'a, vol. i, p. 312.

[2] Really the governor of Ray, Manṣúr ibn Isḥáq ibn Aḥmad. See my translation of the *Chahár Maqála* ("E. J. W. Gibb Memorial" Series, xi, 2, p. 150).

shortly changed colour. Thinking to put an end to his life with this poisonous mixture he consumed the greater part of it, after which he fell into a deep sleep, from which he awoke in a copious perspiration, and, after violent purging, found that he was quit of his dropsy and his appetite had returned.

A third anecdote similar to the last, related by a man named Abú 'Alí 'Umar ibn Yaḥyá al-'Alawí[1], concerns a fellow-pilgrim from Kúfa who suffered from dropsy and was kidnapped with his camel by Arab marauders. One day his captors entered the hut where he was lying, bringing some snakes which they had caught, and which they proceeded to roast and eat after they had cut off their heads and tails. He, hoping that this unaccustomed food would poison him, craved a portion and ate it, when, after experiencing precisely the same symptoms as the sufferer mentioned in the last story, he similarly found himself cured of his sickness.

A fourth anecdote[2] is of a boy who suffered from violent pain and throbbing in the stomach for which no cause or cure could be found, though he was examined by many physicians of Ahwáz in S.W. Persia, a well-known town situated near the once famous medical school of Jundí-Shápúr, of which I spoke in a previous lecture. Finally he was sent home, and there a passing physician, not named, cross-examined him at length and discovered that his ailment dated from a day when he had eaten pomegranates stored in a cow-house. The physician next day brought him broth made with the flesh of a fat puppy, and bade him take as much as he could of it, while refusing to make known its nature. Then he gave him to eat a quantity of melon, and two hours later beer mixed with hot

---

[1] *Al-Faraj*, vol. ii, p. 100.   [2] *Ibid.*, vol. ii, pp. 96–7.

water, after which he informed him how the broth had been prepared. Thereupon the patient was violently sick, and in his vomit the physician presently discovered "a black thing like a large date-stone which moved," and which proved to be a sheep- or cattle-tick which had entered the pomegranate, been accidentally swallowed by the boy, and attached itself to the coats of his stomach, from which, like the leech in a previous anecdote, it was induced to detach itself by being presented with a more attractive substance.

The case of another dropsical patient forms the subject of a fifth of these anecdotes. He was, after being dosed with various drugs, pronounced incurable by the physicians of Baghdád, and thereupon begged that he might be allowed to eat and drink what he pleased, and not, as he expressed it, be "destroyed by dieting." One day he saw a man selling cooked locusts, of which he bought and ate a large quantity. Violent purging followed this repast and lasted three days, at the end of which he was so weak that his life was despaired of, but he gradually recovered and was entirely cured of his dropsy. On the fifth day, being able to walk abroad, he met one of the physicians who had seen him before, and who was amazed at his recovery, about which he questioned him. "These were no ordinary locusts," said the physician, when he had heard the story; "I should like you to point out to me the man who sold them to you." The seller being found and questioned, said that he collected the locusts in a village some miles from Baghdád, whither, for a small reward, he accompanied the physician, who found the locusts in a field in which grew quantities of the herb called *Mádharyún* (identified by Schlimmer and Achundow as *Daphne oleoides*, the Laurel-spurge or Spurge-flax), known to be beneficial in small doses for dropsy, but too dangerous to be commonly prescribed[1]. The double coction which it had undergone in the locusts' bodies had, however, so mitigated its violence that its results had in this case proved wholly beneficial.

Other anecdotes in this book, on which I have not time to dwell, include a cure of apoplexy by flagellation, of pleurisy by a scorpion-bite, and of paralysis by a decoction of colocynth in milk.

The Persian collection of anecdotes to which I alluded above was compiled by Muḥammad 'Awfí about A.D. 1230, and is entitled *Jawámi'u'l-Ḥikáyát wa Lawámi'u'r-Riwáyát*. It is a gigantic work, comprising four volumes, each consisting of twenty-five chapters, and has never yet been published; but I am fortunate enough to possess one complete MS. and another of the first volume. The twentieth chapter of this volume concerns Physicians, and comprises nine anecdotes, four of which are taken from at-Tanúkhí's work "Relief after Distress," described above. In only one of the five new stories is mention made of Rhazes, who is represented as curing a patient of intussusception or obstruction of the intestines by giving him two drachms of quicksilver. In the remaining anecdotes there is little worth notice except one aphorism and one story. The aphorism, uttered by an unnamed physician to a patient, is as follows: "Know that I and thou and the disease are three factors mutually antagonistic. If thou wilt side with me, not neglecting what I enjoin on thee and

[1] See the *Qánún* of Avicenna (ed. Rome, 1593), p. 205, and the Latin translation (Venice, 1544), p. 147, where two drachms of this "Mezereon" are said to be fatal to man. In the *Burhán-i-Qáṭi'* and the *Farhang-i-Násirí* the form *Mázaryún* (with ج instead of ز) is given.

refraining from such food as I shall forbid thee, then we shall be two against one and will overcome the disease." The story, which concerns Aristotle and an Indian physician named Sarbát or Sarnáb—who came to him incognito as a disciple in order to study his methods, but revealed himself at a critical stage in the trephining of a patient—is a very absurd one, about a millipede or ear-wig (*hazár-páy* or *gúsh-khúrak*) which entered the patient's ear and attached itself to his brain. The interesting point in it is that, before beginning the operation, Aristotle "gave him a drug so that he became unconscious." I have only met with one earlier reference to anaesthesia in Persian literature, namely the well-known passage in the *Sháh-náma*, or "Book of Kings," of Firdawsí[1] (composed early in the eleventh century of our era) describing the Caesarean section practised on Rúdába, the mother of Rustam, at the time of his birth, though in this case wine was the agent used to produce unconsciousness, while the operator was a *Múbadh* or Zoroastrian priest.

Another Persian book, entitled *Chahár Maqála* (the "Four Discourses"), and composed about A.D. 1155 by a court-poet of Samarqand named Niẓámí-i-'Arúdí, affords more copious material for our present purpose than either of the books mentioned above. The author treats of four classes of experts whom he considers indispensable at a properly constituted court, to wit Secretaries of State, Poets, Astrologers and Physicians; for, as he observes with propriety, the business of kings cannot be conducted without competent secretaries; their triumphs and victories will not be immortalized without eloquent poets; their enterprises will not succeed

---

[1] Ed. Turner Macan, vol. i, pp. 162–3.

unless undertaken at seasons adjudged propitious by sagacious astrologers; while health, the basis of all happiness and activity, can only be secured by the services of able and trustworthy physicians. Each Discourse, therefore, deals with one of these classes, in the order given above, and, after some preliminary remarks on the qualifications requisite for success in the profession in question, gives a number of anecdotes (about ten as a rule) illustrating the author's views. These are of special value as being for the greater part derived from his own recollections and experience. Twenty years ago I published a complete translation of this work in the *Journal of the Royal Asiatic Society*[1]; ten years later a critical text with Persian notes was prepared by a learned Persian friend of mine, Mírzá Muḥammad Khán of Qazwín, and published in the " E. J. W. Gibb Memorial " Series[2]; and I am now engaged on a revised and annotated translation in which special attention has been given to the medical anecdotes. The fact that this book is now reasonably accessible renders it unnecessary for me to speak at greater length about it, and I shall confine myself to a few remarks on the Fourth Discourse dealing with Physicians.

"The physician," says our author, "should be of tender disposition, of wise and gentle nature, and more especially an acute observer, capable of benefiting everyone by accurate diagnosis, that is to say, by rapid deduction of the unknown from the known. And no

---

[1] July and October, 1899. The separate reprint, now exhausted, comprises, with the Index, 139 pages.

[2] It is vol. xi of this series, and was published in 1910. The revised and annotated translation, now in the Press, will constitute vol. xi, 2, of the same series.

physician can be of tender disposition if he fails to recognize the nobility of man; nor of philosophical nature unless he be acquainted with Logic; nor an acute observer unless he be strengthened by God's guidance; and he who is not an accurate observer will not arrive at a correct understanding of the cause of any ailment."

After developing this thesis, and relating the case of a sick man healed by prayer, the author gives an instructive list of the books which should be read by the aspirant to medical science, which range from the *Aphorisms* of Hippocrates and the Sixteen Treatises of Galen to the great "Thesaurus" of Medicine compiled in Persian for the Sháh of Khwárazm, or Khiva, by Sayyid Isma'íl of Jurján only twenty or thirty years earlier. "But," he concludes, "if the student desires to be independent of other works, he may rest satisfied with the *Qánún* of Avicenna," whom he puts second only to Aristotle, and praises in the highest terms as the only thinker during fifteen centuries who has won to the inmost essence of the Aristotelian philosophy and travelled the road of his great predecessor's pre-eminence.

The anecdotes which follow are of a somewhat different type from those we have hitherto considered; we find none of those grotesque stories of abnormal parasitic invasion, or of the therapeutic virtues of vipers and locusts. On the other hand elementary methods of psychotherapeusis form the subject-matter of no less than four of the narratives, and several of these have passed into general Persian literature, even poetry, and have thus attained considerable notoriety. We may take first two of the best known, wherein the emotions of anger and shame are employed respectively in the treatment of rheumatic affections of the joints.

The great physician Rhazes was summoned to Transoxiana to attend the Amír Manṣúr, who was suffering from a rheumatic affection of the joints which baffled all his medical attendants. On arriving at the Oxus, Rhazes was so much alarmed at its size and the small and fragile appearance of the boat in which he was invited to embark that he declined to proceed further, until the King's messengers bound him hand and foot, threw him into the boat, and carried him across by force, though otherwise they treated him with the utmost respect and even apologized for the use of violence, begging him to bear them no grudge. Rhazes assured them that he harboured no resentment and explained the motive of his resistance. "I know," said he, "that every year many thousand persons cross the Oxus safely, but, had I chanced to be drowned, people would have said, 'What a fool Muhammad ibn Zakariyyá was to expose himself to this risk of his own free will.' But, being carried across by force, had I then perished people would have pitied, not blamed me."

On reaching Bukhárá he tried various methods of treatment on the Amír without success. Finally he said to him, "To-morrow I shall try a new treatment, but it will cost you the best horse and best mule in your stables." The Amír agreed and placed the animals at his disposal. Next day Rhazes brought the Amír to a hot bath outside the city, tied up the horse and the mule, saddled and bridled, outside, and entered the hot room of the bath alone with his patient, to whom he administered douches of hot water and a draught which he had prepared "till such time" says the narrator, "as the humours in his joints were matured. Then he went out, put on his clothes, and, taking a knife in his hand, came in, and stood for a while reviling the Amír, saying, 'Thou didst order me to be bound and cast into the boat, and didst conspire against my life. If I do not destroy thee as a punishment for this, my name is not Muḥammad ibn Zakariyyá!' The Amír was furious, and, partly from anger, partly from fear, sprang to his feet." Rhazes at once fled from the bath to where his servant was awaiting him outside with the horse and the mule, rode off at full gallop, and did not pause in his flight until he had crossed the Oxus and reached Merv, whence he wrote to the Amír as follows[1]:

"May the life of the King be prolonged in health and authority! Agreeably to my undertaking I treated you to the best of my ability. There was, however, a deficiency in the natural caloric, and this treatment would have been unduly protracted, so I abandoned it in favour of psychotherapeusis (*'iláj-i-nafsání*), and, when the peccant humours had undergone sufficient coction in the bath, I deliberately provoked you in order to increase the natural caloric, which thus gained sufficient strength to dissolve the already softened humours. But henceforth it is inexpedient that we should meet."

The Amír, having recovered from his anger, was delighted to find himself restored to health and freedom of movement, and caused search to be made everywhere for the physician, but in vain, until on the seventh day his servant returned with the horse and mule and the letter cited above. As Rhazes persisted in his resolution not to return, the Amír rewarded him with a robe of honour, a cloak, a turban, arms, a male and female slave, and a horse fully caparisoned, and further assigned to

---

[1] I have slightly abridged and otherwise modified the letter, of which the literal translation will be found on p. 117 of the separate reprint of my translation in the *J. R. A. S.* for 1899, and on p. 84 of the forthcoming revised translation.

him a yearly pension of 2000 gold *dínárs* and 200 ass-loads of corn.

This anecdote is cited in a well-known Persian ethical work, the *Akhláq-i-Jalálí*, composed three hundred years later than the *Chahár Maqála*. In the other anecdote which I place in the same category the patient is a woman in the King's household who, while bending down to lay the table, is attacked by a sudden "rheumatic swelling of the joints," and is unable to assume an erect posture. The King's physician (not named), being commanded to cure her, and having no medicaments at hand, has recourse to "psychic treatment" (*tadbír-i-nafsání*) and, by removing first her veil and then her skirt, calls to his aid the emotion of shame, whereby, in the author's words, "a flush of heat was produced within her which dissolved the rheumatic humour," so that she stood upright completely cured. This story is retold by the great poet Jámí, who flourished about the end of the fifteenth century, in his *Silsilatu'dh-Dhahab* or "Chain of Gold," but, much more important, it has been found by Mírzá Muḥammad Khán in a manuscript of Avicenna's rare and unpublished *Kitábu'l-Mabda' wa'l-Ma'ád* (the "Book of the Origin and the Return"), whence the author of the *Chahár Maqála* avowedly took it[1]. Avicenna, therefore, evidently believed the story, though he too omits the name of the physician, only stating that he was in the service of one of the Sámánid rulers, who flourished in Khurásán and Transoxiana in the tenth century.

Of both the two next anecdotes Avicenna is again the hero. When in his flight from Maḥmúd of Ghazna he came incognito to Jurján or Gurgán (the ancient

---

[1] See p. 73 of the text and p. 242 of the notes in vol. xi of the "E. J. W. Gibb Memorial" Series.

Hyrcania) by the Caspian Sea, a relative of the ruler of that province lay sick of a malady which baffled all the local doctors. Avicenna, though his identity was then unknown, was invited to give his opinion, and, after examining the patient, requested the collaboration of someone who knew all the districts and towns of the province, and who repeated their names while Avicenna kept his finger on the patient's pulse. At the mention of a certain town he felt a flutter in the pulse. "Now," said he, "I need someone who knows all the houses, streets and quarters of this town." Again when a certain street was mentioned the same phenomenon was repeated, and once again when the names of the inhabitants of a certain household were enumerated. Then Avicenna said, "It is finished. This lad is in love with such-and-such a girl, who lives in such-and-such a house, in such-and-such a street, in such-and-such a quarter of such-and-such a town; and the girl's face is the patient's cure." So the marriage was solemnized at a fortunate hour chosen by Avicenna, and thus the cure was completed.

For this story again, or at least for its essential feature, we have the best authority, namely Avicenna's own statement in the *Qánún*[1] in the section devoted to Love, which is classed under cerebral or mental diseases, together with somnolence, insomnia, amnesia, mania, hydrophobia, melancholia, and the like. In the Latin translation[2] this section is hardly recognizable under the title *De Ilixi*, with *alhasch* as a marginal variant, both these monstrosities being intended to represent

---

[1] See p. 316 of the Arabic text printed at Rome in A.D. 1593. Ibn Abí Uṣaybi'a (vol. ii, p. 128) relates very similar anecdotes of Galen and of Rashídu'd-Dín Abú Ḥalíqa.

[2] Venice, 1544, f. 208 *b*.

the Arabic *al-'Ishq*, "Love." After describing the symptoms, and especially the irregularities of the pulse, Avicenna says:

"And hereby it is possible to arrive at the identity of the beloved person, if the patient will not reveal it, such knowledge affording one means of treatment. The device whereby this may be effected is that many names should be mentioned and repeated while the finger is retained on the pulse, and when it becomes very irregular and almost ceases, one should then repeat the process. I have tried this method repeatedly, and have discovered the name of the beloved. Then, in like manner, mention the streets, dwellings, arts, crafts, families and countries, joining each one with the name of the beloved, and all the time feeling the pulse, so that when it alters on the mention of any one thing several times, you will infer from this all particulars about the beloved as regards name, appearance and occupation. We have ourselves tried this plan, and have thereby arrived at knowledge which was valuable. Then, if you can discover no cure except to unite the two in such wise as is sanctioned by religion and law, you will do this. We have seen cases where health and strength were completely restored and flesh regained, after the patient had become greatly attenuated and suffered from severe chronic diseases and protracted accesses of fever from lack of strength resulting from excessive love, when he was accorded union with his beloved......in a very short time, so that we were astonished thereat and realized the subordination of [human] nature to mental imaginations."

We find a further allusion to this treatment in a later medical encyclopaedia to which I have already alluded, the *Dhakhíra-i-Khwárazmsháhí*, composed between

A.D. 1111 and 1136, and notable as the first great system of Medicine written in the Persian instead of in the Arabic language. Here also the author, Sayyid Isma'íl of Jurján, after repeating the substance of Avicenna's directions, adds: "Master Abú 'Alí (*i.e.* Avicenna), upon whom be God's mercy, says, 'I have tried this plan and have so discovered who the beloved object was,'" and appends a fairly close translation of Avicenna's concluding words as to the rapid recovery of the patient when his desire is fulfilled.

Rather more than a hundred years later, in the middle of the thirteenth century, the great mystical poet Jalálu'd-Dín Rúmí, who may be called the Dante of Persia, made this theme the subject of the allegorical anecdote which comes at the beginning of his celebrated *Mathnawí*. This anecdote describes how a king while hunting saw a very beautiful girl, fell in love with her, and married her. To his great distress she forthwith sickened, nor could the physicians summoned to her bedside alleviate her malady or assuage her suffering, because, when assuring the king that they could cure her, they omitted the saving clause (*istithná*) " Please God." Hence all their drugs produced the opposite effects to those intended and desired ; oxymel (*sirkangabín*) only increased her biliousness, and myrobolans (*halíla*) desiccated instead of relaxing. Finally, in answer to the king's prayers, a "divine physician" (*ṭabíb-i-iláhí*) appears, and, after a careful examination of the patient, announces that the treatment hitherto pursued has been wholly mischievous and based on a wrong diagnosis. He then asks to be left alone with the patient and proceeds to question her about the towns where she has previously lived, since, he explains, treatment varies according to place of origin or sojourn. While talking to her about her past history he keeps his finger on her pulse, but observes no sign of emotion until Samarqand is mentioned, and again later at the name of the Sar-i-pul or "Bridge-end" quarter and the street called Ghátafar[1]. In short he finally discovers, in precisely the way indicated by Avicenna, that she is in love with a certain goldsmith living in that quarter of Samarqand. Thereupon, having reassured her and promised her recovery, he instructs the king to send messengers to Samarqand to invite the goldsmith to his court and offer him handsome remuneration. The unsuspecting goldsmith comes blithely, flattered by the king's gracious words, fine gifts and fair promises, and on his arrival, by the "divine physician's" instructions, is married to the girl, who in the course of six months recovers her health and good looks. Then the physician begins to administer to the goldsmith a slow poison which causes him to become "ugly, displeasing and sallow," so that the girl wearies of him before his death, which is not long delayed, places her once more at the disposal of the king, whose bride she now becomes. Into the allegorical meaning of this outwardly immoral story I have not time to enter now, but this purely literary use of medical material indirectly borrowed from Avicenna himself appears to me to be of considerable interest.

From the "Four Discourses" I shall only cite one more anecdote, of which again Avicenna is the hero. A certain prince of the House of Buwayh was afflicted with melancholia and suffered from the delusion that he was a cow. "Every day," says the author, "he would low like a cow, causing annoyance to everyone, and

---

[1] This actually exists. See V. Zhukovski's Развалины Стараго Мерва, p. 171, n. 1.

crying, 'Kill me, so that a good stew may be prepared from my flesh'; until matters reached such a pass that he would eat nothing, while the physicians were unable to do him any good." Finally Avicenna, who was at this time acting as prime minister to 'Alá'u'd-Dawla ibn Kákúya, was persuaded to take the case in hand, which in spite of the pressure of public and private business, political, scientific and literary, with which he was overwhelmed, he consented to do. First of all he sent a message to the patient bidding him be of good cheer because the butcher was coming to slaughter him, whereat, we are told, the sick man rejoiced. Some time afterwards Avicenna, holding a knife in his hand, entered the sick-room, saying, "Where is this cow, that I may kill it?" The patient lowed like a cow to indicate where he was. By Avicenna's orders he was laid on the ground bound hand and foot. Avicenna then felt him all over and said, "He is too lean, and not ready to be killed; he must be fattened." Then they offered him suitable food, of which he now partook eagerly, and gradually he gained strength, got rid of his delusion, and was completely cured. The narrator concludes, "All wise men will perceive that one cannot heal by such methods of treatment save by virtue of pre-eminent intelligence, perfect science and unerring acumen." This anecdote also has been versified by Jámí in his "Chain of Gold" (*Silsilatu'dh-Dhahab*) composed in A.D. 1485, three hundred and thirty years after the "Four Discourses," but I can find no allusion to any such method of treatment in the article on Melancholia in the *Qánún* of Avicenna.

Before leaving this topic, I must refer to an anecdote given by the poet Nizámí in his "Treasury of Secrets" (*Makhzanu'l-Asrár*), where suggestion is employed not to heal but to destroy. This story relates how the rivalry between two court physicians finally reached such a point that they challenged one another to a duel or ordeal by poison, it being agreed that each should take a poison supplied by his antagonist, of which he should then endeavour to counteract the effects by a suitable antidote. The first prepared a poisonous draught "the fierceness of which would have melted black stone"; his rival drained the cup and at once took an antidote which rendered it innocuous. It was now his turn, and he picked a rose from the garden, breathed an incantation over it, and bade his antagonist smell it, whereupon the latter at once fell down dead. That his death was due simply to fear and not to any poisonous or magical property of the rose is clearly indicated by the poet:

دشمن از آن گُل که فسون خوان بداد ،
ترس بدو چیره شد و جان بداد ،
آن بعلاج از تنِ خود زهر بُرد ،
وین بیکی گُل ز توهّم بمُرد ،

"Through this rose which the spell-breather had given him
Fear overmastered the foe and he gave up the ghost.
That one by treatment expelled the poison from his body,
While this one died of a rose from fear."

I have little doubt that suggestion played an important part in Arabian Medicine, and that wider reading in Arabic and Persian books (often sadly discursive and unsystematic, and, of course, never provided with indexes) would yield a much richer harvest in this field. But the people of the East have much of the child's love of the marvellous; they like their kings to be immensely great and powerful, their queens and princesses incomparably

beautiful, their ministers or *wazírs* abnormally sagacious, and their physicians superhumanly discerning and
resourceful. This unbounded faith, which is in fact most
embarrassing to one who practises medicine in the East,
is sustained and extended by such sensational stories as
I have cited. Rhazes did this, they will tell you, and
Avicenna that, and are not you, the heir of all the ages,
greater than these, nay, even than Hippocrates and
Galen? Yet the genuine case-book of Rhazes, of which,
almost alone in Arabic literature, a fragment has happily
been preserved to us in a Bodleian MS.[1] mentioned in a
former lecture, altogether lacks this sensational quality,
and it is to the credit of that great physician that he
should have chosen to record precisely those cases which
puzzled him at first or baffled him altogether.

In the opening lecture of this course I explained
that, while the Golden Age of Islamic or Arabian
literature and science was the first century or two of
the 'Abbásid Caliphate of Baghdád (*i.e.* from A.D. 750
onwards), a high level of culture continued to be maintained until the awful catastrophe of the Mongol or
Tartar invasion of the thirteenth century inflicted on it
a blow from which it has never recovered. The Caliphate
was overthrown and its metropolis sacked and laid waste
in A.D. 1258, and though the surviving scholars of the
younger generation carried on the sound tradition of
scholarship for a while longer, there is, broadly speaking,
a difference not only of degree but of kind between
the literary and scientific work done before and after
the thirteenth century throughout the lands of Islám.
Medicine and history owed their comparative immunity
to the desire of the savage conquerors for health and

---

[1] **Marsh 156**, ff. 239 *b*–246 *a*. See pp. 50–53 *supra*.

fame, and in the next lecture I shall have to speak of at least one writer who flourished even as late as the fourteenth century. Of course from that time to the present day there has been no lack of medical literature of a sort: some idea of the number of medical works composed in Persian alone may be gathered from Adolf Fonahn's *Zur Quellenkunde der Persischen Medizin*, published at Leipzig in 1910. The author of this excellent and painstaking book enumerates over 400 Persian works (very few of which have been published) dealing entirely or partly with medical subjects, and adds a very useful bibliography[1] and short biographical notices of 25 of the most notable Persian physicians[2] and writers on Medicine who flourished from the end of the tenth to the beginning of the eighteenth century, excluding, however, such men as Rhazes, " Haly Abbas " and Avicenna who, though Persian by race, wrote in Arabic. This vernacular medical literature of Persia remains almost unexplored, nor could it, as a rule, be explored with advantage until a much more thorough examination of the older Arabic literature has been effected. A thorough knowledge of the contents of the *Ḥáwí* or "Continens," the *Kitábu'l-Malikí* or "Liber Regius" and the *Qánún* of Avicenna would be necessary in order to decide whether any substantial addition to, or modification of, these classics was effected by the later writers. Of one great Persian system of Medicine, compiled in the twelfth century, the *Dhakhíra-i-Khwárazmsháhí*, which good fortune has rendered accessible to me in several manuscripts, I propose to speak in the next lecture. Only two other Persian medical works have hitherto, so far as I know, attracted much attention in Europe—Abú Mansúr

---

[1] pp. 135–140.　　　　[2] pp. 129–134.

Muwaffaq of Herát's *Materia Medica*, composed about
A.D. 950, and the illustrated *Anatomy* of Manṣúr ibn
Muḥammad, composed in A.D. 1396. The oldest known
Persian manuscript in Europe, copied by the poet Asadí
in A.D. 1055, is the unique original of the former, and
was produced at Vienna by Dr F. R. Seligmann in
1859 in a most beautiful and artistic edition on which
excellent work has been done by Abdul-Chalig Achundow, Dr Paul Horn and Professor Jolly. The anatomical
diagrams contained in the latter have especially attracted
the attention of Dr Karl Sudhoff, who published them
from the India Office MS. in *Studien zur Geschichte der
Medizin*[1], and who has suggested that they represent
an ancient tradition going back, perhaps, even to the
Alexandrian School. Of this work I have recently acquired two MSS. in which some of the illustrations show
variations which may prove of interest.

Before concluding this lecture I may add a few
words about the introduction of modern European
Medicine into the Muslim East, where the old system,
which we call Arabian and the Muslims Greek (*Ṭibb-i-
Yúnání*), still maintains itself, while slowly giving
ground, especially in Persia and India. When I was at
Ṭihrán in 1887 Dr Tholozon, physician to His late
Majesty Náṣiru'd-Dín Sháh, kindly enabled me to attend the meetings of the *Majlis-i-Ṣiḥḥat*, or Council of
Public Health, in the Persian capital, and a majority of
the physicians present at that time knew no medicine
but that of Avicenna. Since that time a good many
young Persians (though far fewer than one would wish)
have come to Europe to study, but even in the middle
of the nineteenth century much was being done by such
men as Dr Polak, the Austrian, and Dr Schlimmer, the

[1] Heft 4, Leipzig, 1908.

Dutchman, who went out to Persia to organize the new Polytechnic and Military Colleges. Dr Schlimmer's *Terminologie Médico-Pharmaceutique et Anthropologique Française-Persane*, lithographed at Ṭihrán in 1874, is, indeed,- invaluable to students of Oriental Medicine by reason of the mass of information it contains and the careful identifications of the Persian names of plants, drugs and diseases. One of the earliest books printed in Persia with movable types was a treatise on inoculation for small-pox (which I have not seen) published at Tabríz in 1825[1]. This very same year marks the introduction of modern medical science into Egypt by Clot Bey and other French scientists invited thither by the Khedive Muḥammad 'Alí, and the establishment of the hospital at Abú Za'bal near Heliopolis, which was transferred a year later to its present site at Qaṣru'l-'Ayní. Egyptian students had been sent to Italy in 1813 and 1816 and to England in 1818 to study military and naval science, ship-building, printing and mechanics, but the first medical students seem to have been sent to Paris, no doubt at the instigation of Clot Bey, in 1826. An excellent account of this latest revival of science (*an-Nahḍatu'l-Akhíra*, as it is called in Arabic) is given by that indefatigable writer the late Jurjí Zaydán, a Christian Syrian domiciled in Egypt, in his *History of Arabic Literature*[2], published in Cairo in 1911–14. To speak of it in detail would lead me too far from my subject, but two points connected with its history have a certain bearing on the revival of Greek learning in the East in the eighth century, which I dealt with in my first lecture last year. I spoke there of the

---

[1] See E. G. Browne's *Press and Poetry of Modern Persia* (Cambridge, 1914), p. 7.

[2] *Ta'ríkhu Ádábi 'l-Lughati 'l-'Arabiyya*, vol. iv, pp. 24 *et seqq.*

prejudice against dissection; and it is interesting to note that Clot Bey's struggles against this same prejudice brought him within measurable distance of assassination[1]. I also observed that while some Greek books were translated directly into Arabic for the Caliphs of Baghdád, in many cases there was an intermediate translation into Syriac. So in the "latest revival," which took place at Cairo a thousand years later, we learn[2] that one of the most skilful translators, Ḥunayn or Yuḥanná 'Anḥúrí (whom we may well entitle the second Ḥunayn or Johannitius), "was weak in French but well grounded in Italian, from which he used to translate into Arabic. So when the book was written in French it was first translated for him into Italian, from which he translated it into Arabic." Whether made directly or indirectly from the original, the first Arabic translation before it went to press commonly passed through the hands of an editor or "corrector" (quite distinct from the reader of the press) who was a good Arabic scholar, knowing something of the science in question and its terminology, but ignorant of any European language, and who gave the book a proper literary form. A similar procedure, according to Dr Lucien Leclerc, characterized the translation of Arabic scientific books into Latin in the Middle Ages[3].

How aptly does Abu 'l-'Alá al-Ma'arrí liken time to a long poem, in which the rhyme, metre and rhythm never vary, though the same rhyming word is never repeated.

[1] See his *Aperçu général sur l'Égypte*, vol. ii, p. 415 (Paris, 1840).

[2] p. 190 of Zaydán's work mentioned in the last note but one.

[3] *Histoire de la Médecine Arabe*, vol. ii, pp. 344 and 345.

و كَأَنَّها هٰذا الزمانُ قصيدةٌ،   ما اَضْطُرَّ شاعِرُها الى ايطائِها،

"Die Zeit, die ewig dahin rollt,   ist wie ein Gedicht:
Doch denselben Reim wiederholt   der Dichter nicht[1]."

So says the historian Ibn Khaldún, "The Past more closely resembles the Future than water resembles water."

الماضى أشبه بالآتى من الماء بالماء،

[1] A. von Kremer's *Culturgeschichte des Orients*, vol. ii, p. 390, and the *Z. D. M. G.*, vol. xxx, p. 44. Dr R. A. Nicholson, in his recently published *Studies in Islamic Poetry* (Cambridge, 1921, p. 59), translates this same verse thus:

> *"And the Maker infinite,*
> *Whose poem is Time,*
> *He need not weave in it*
> *A forced stale rhyme."*

LECTURE IV

THE brief survey of the history and development of Arabian Medicine which I have attempted in the last three lectures, and which I must conclude to-day, has necessarily been somewhat severely limited by considerations of time; and I have been obliged to confine myself for the most part to the period and realms of the 'Abbásid Caliphs, that is the eighth to the thirteenth centuries of our era, and the regions of Mesopotamia and Persia. I regret that I am compelled to exclude from this survey the brilliant civilization developed in Spain and the West under Arab dominion; but, lest you should forget it, or think that I have forgotten it, I must at least mention a few of the most illustrious names associated with Moorish Medicine. In the tenth century Cordova produced the greatest surgeon of the Arab race, Abu'l-Qásim az-Zahráwí, known to medieval Europe as Abulcasis (or even Albucasis) and Alsaharavius, with whom was contemporary the court-physician Ibn Juljul, whose *Lives of the Physicians and Philosophers* is unhappily lost. "Aben Guefit," properly Ibnu'l-Wáfid, of Toledo, and Ibnu'l-Jazzár of Qayruwán in Tunisia, who sought relaxation from his professional labours in piracy on the high seas, belong to a slightly later generation. The twelfth century produced the famous Averroes (Ibn Rushd) of Cordova, who was, however, more notable as a philosopher than as a physician; Avenzoar (Ibn Zuhr) of Seville; and the famous Jewish scholar Maimonides (Músá ibn Maymún), also of Cordova, who finally became court-physician to Saladin in Egypt. One other name of the thirteenth century which must on no account be omitted is the great botanist Ibnu'l-

Bayṭár of Malaga, a worthy successor of Dioscorides, who travelled widely through Greece, Asia Minor and Egypt in search of medicinal herbs, and whose works on Materia Medica have been made known in Europe by Sontheimer and Leclerc. In the transmission of the Arabian system of Medicine to Europe, Spain and N.W. Africa, as you are well aware, played the chief part; and in particular Toledo, where men like Gerard of Cremona and Michael Scot[1] sought the knowledge which they afterwards conveyed to Christian Europe.

Turning now once more to Persia, the twelfth century is remarkable for the development of a vernacular medical and scientific literature of which only scanty traces are found in earlier times. Arabic, still the chief vehicle of theological and philosophical thought throughout the lands of Islám, as Latin was in medieval Europe, had hitherto been used almost exclusively even by the great Persian physicians Rhazes, Haly Abbas and Avicenna of whom I have spoken. But in the early part of the twelfth century there came to the court of Khwárazm or Khiva a physician named Zaynu'd-Dín Isma'íl of Jurján (Hyrcania), who wrote several medical works, of which the most important and by far the largest is entitled, in honour of the ruler to whom it was dedicated, *Dhakhíra-i-Khwárazmsháhí*, or the "Thesaurus" of the King of Khwárazm. This work, which rivals if it does not exceed in scope and size the *Qánún* of Avicenna, remains unpublished, though I believe that a lithographed Urdú translation is still in use in India. I possess, besides several isolated volumes, some transcribed in the thirteenth and fourteenth centuries, one

----

[1] The period at which Gerard of Cremona (b. 1114, d. 1187) visited Toledo is uncertain. Michael Scot was there in 1217.

complete manuscript of this encyclopaedic work comprising 1403 pages measuring 12×8 inches and each
comprising 27 lines. The book cannot contain much
fewer than 450,000 words; and as the writing is by no
means clear, the text far from correct, and there are, of
course, neither head-lines nor indexes, it will be easily
understood that the perusal of it is somewhat laborious.
It is, however, elaborately divided and subdivided,
primarily into nine volumes, with a tenth supplementary
volume on Materia Medica, and secondarily into in-
numerable Discourses (*Guftár*), Parts (*Juz'*) and
Chapters (*Báb*), of which, with the help of another
almost complete manuscript belonging to the Cambridge
University Library, I have succeeded in making an ex-
haustive table. I may note that the Library of this
College possesses a very fine old twelfth century manuscript[1] of part of the sixth volume, which treats of local
diseases *a capite ad calcem*, including all six chapters of
the eighth Discourse on diseases of the heart, and part
of the thirteenth Discourse dealing with dropsy.

The same author composed several smaller medical
works, all in Persian, namely the "Aims of Medicine"
(*Aghrád-i-Ṭibb*), the "Remembrancer" (*Yádgár*) on
Materia Medica and Pharmacy, and the *Khuffí-i-'Alá'í*
written in two elongated volumes to be carried by the
traveller one in each of his riding-boots (*khuff*), whence
its name. All these are described by Fonahn in his useful work *Zur Quellenkunde der Persischen Medizin*, and
all are recommended by the author of the "Four Discourses" (*Chahár Maqála*), written only twenty years
after the death of Zaynu'd-Dín Isma'íl. Of the "Thesaurus," by which term I shall henceforth denote the
Dhakhíra-i-Khwárazmsháhí, I shall have a good deal

[1] Marked A. 27.

more to say, but first I will complete my literary survey down to the Mongol period, beyond which I do not propose to go.

The thirteenth century is remarkable for the number of excellent biographical works in Arabic which it produced. First, as containing only medical biographies, I will mention the '*Uyúnu'l-Anbá fí Ṭabaqátí'l-Aṭibbá* ("Sources of Information on the Classes of Physicians"), compiled by Ibn Abí Uṣaybi'a at Damascus in A.D. 1245, and printed at Cairo in two volumes in 1882. Then there is the *Ta'ríkhu'l-Ḥukamá*, a biographical dictionary of philosophers and physicians composed by al-Qifṭí, a native of Upper Egypt, a great lover and collector of books, who combined piety with tolerance and was generous in his help to other scholars, and who died at the age of 76 in A.D. 1248. The text of this valuable work, edited by Dr Julius Lippert, was published at Leipzig in 1903. Another similar but rather earlier work by Shahrazúrí exists in two recensions, one Arabic and one Persian, but is rare and remains unpublished. The great biographical dictionary of Ibn Khallikán, begun in Cairo in A.D. 1256 and finished in the same city in A.D. 1274, is accessible to the English reader in the translation of the Baron McGuckin de Slane, and, though more general in its scope, contains the lives of several physicians of note. The geographer Yáqút, who flourished about the same time, also wrote a biographical dictionary, of which five volumes have been edited by Professor Margoliouth, but this deals chiefly with men of letters. Lastly, mention must be made of the Christian physician, philosopher, theologian and historian, Abu'l-Faraj Gregorius, better known as Bar Hebraeus, who died at the age of 60 in A.D. 1286, and whom the late Dr Wright[1] has described as "one of the most learned and versatile men that Syria ever produced." He wrote chiefly in Syriac, but at the end of his life, at the request of some Muslim friends at Marágha in N.W. Persia, he produced an Arabic recension of the first or political portion of his great Universal History "enriched with many references to Muhammadan writers and literature which are wanting in the Syriac" original. Being himself a physician of note, enjoying in a high degree the favour and confidence of the Mongol rulers of Persia, he naturally devotes a good deal of attention in his history to medical matters. This book was edited with a Latin translation by Pocock in A.D. 1663, and another excellent edition with full indexes was published by the Catholic Press at Beyrout in A.D. 1890.

What we chiefly lack in order to form a picture of the practice of Medicine in the lands of Islám during the Middle Ages is some account of the actual administration of the hospitals founded in considerable numbers in the more important towns by pious benefactors. About the actual buildings, indeed, we find information in the narratives of travellers like Ibn Baṭúṭa (fourteenth century) and the descriptions of topographers like al-Maqrízí (fifteenth century), who gives particulars as to the history, situation and structure of five hospitals in Cairo[2]. The oldest of these was that founded by Aḥmad ibn Ṭúlún about A.D. 873; the most important that founded by Qalá'ún about A.D. 1284 and called "the great hospital of al-Manṣúr" (*al-Máristán al-Kabír al-Manṣúrí*). It was founded by Qalá'ún

[1] *Syriac Literature* (London, 1894), p. 265. For a list of his medical works, see p. 252 of the same.

[2] *Khiṭaṭ* (Buláq, 1853), vol. ii, pp. 405–8. See also E. W. Lane's *Cairo Fifty Years Ago* (London, 1896), pp. 92–4.

al-Malik al-Manṣúr in fulfilment of a vow which he made some years earlier when he was cured of a severe attack of colic at Damascus by physicians attached to the hospital founded in that city by Núru'd-Dín, under whom the great Saladdin first served. The endowments amounted to a million *dirhams* annually; it was open to all sick persons, rich or poor, male or female, and contained wards for women as well as men, and female as well as male attendants were appointed for the care of the patients. One large ward was set apart for fevers, one for ophthalmic cases, one for surgical cases and one for dysentery and kindred ailments. There were also kitchens, lecture-rooms, store-rooms for drugs and apparatus, a dispensary, and rooms for the medical officers. It is worth noting that the word *Máristán*, used throughout these books for a hospital, is a corruption of the Persian word *Bímáristán*, which signifies in that language "a place for the sick." It has now been replaced in Egypt by the purely Arabic word *Mustashfá*, meaning "a place where health is sought," while *Máristán* has come to be used in the sense of a mad-house. From the first certain chambers or cells were set apart in these hospitals for lunatics, and Maqrízí tells us how Aḥmad ibn Ṭúlún, the founder of the oldest hospital in Cairo, used to visit it daily until a lunatic begged a pomegranate of him, and then, instead of eating it, threw it at him with such violence that it burst and spoiled his clothes, after which he would never again visit the hospital. Lane, in his *Cairo Fifty Years Ago* (pp. 92–4), gives a pitiful account of the lunatics he saw in the Bímáristán of Qalá'ún when he visited it; while Clot Bey, in his *Aperçu général sur l'Égypte*[1], draws a deplorable picture of the state of

---

[1] Paris, 1840, vol. ii, pp. 382 *et seqq.*

Medicine in that country at the beginning of the nineteenth century.

A very valuable, I believe unique, Persian manuscript which I recently acquired from the library of the late Sir Albert Houtum-Schindler, who during his long residence in Persia had gained more knowledge of that country in all its aspects than anyone now living possesses, throws some light incidentally on the state of Medicine there in the early fourteenth century. One of the most learned men and scholarly writers of that period was the physician Rashídu'd-Dín Faḍlu'lláh, born in A.D. 1247 at Hamadán, where Avicenna is buried. He became court-physician to the Mongol ruler Abáqá, whose successor Gházán, a convert to Islám, formed so high an opinion of him that he appointed him Prime Minister in A.D. 1295. During the twenty-two years for which he held this high and perilous post (for it was quite exceptional for the Minister of a Mongol sovereign to die a natural death) he enjoyed enormous wealth and power, which he used in the most beneficent manner for the foundation of colleges, hospitals and libraries, the endowment of learning, and the encouragement of scholars. On the beautiful quarter which he founded at Tabríz and named after himself *Rab'-i-Rashídí* he lavished endless care, not only adorning it with noble buildings consecrated to pious and learned uses, but drawing thither by his bounty the greatest scholars, the most eminent professional men, and the most skilful artisans of the time from all parts of the world. The extraordinary and minute precautions which he took to perpetuate and diffuse the learning stored in the incomparable libraries of the *Rab'-i-Rashídí* are fully detailed by Quatremère in the Introduction to his *Histoire des Mongols*. Alas, that these precautions in the event proved vain, for when, in July 1318, he finally fell a victim to the intrigues of envious rivals and was put to death, the beautiful suburb on which he had lavished so much thought, care and wealth was utterly wrecked and plundered!

Such in brief was the man who at the height of his power preferred to call himself "Rashíd the physician" rather than indulge in the high-sounding titles of a grandiloquent age; and the manuscript of which I have spoken contains a collection of some fifty of his letters, addressed to many different people on many different subjects, collected and arranged by his secretary Muḥammad of Abarqúh. My friend Muḥammad Shafí', now Professor of Arabic at the Oriental College, Lahore, was good enough to make an abstract of this precious volume, condensing or omitting the precepts and platitudes with which many of the letters are filled, but devoting particular attention to those which contain matters of interest, and especially of medical or pharmaceutical interest. These, ten in number, I propose briefly to discuss, taking them in the order in which they occur in the manuscript.

No. 18 (ff. 34*b*–36*b*), addressed to Khwája 'Alá'u'd-Dín Hindú, demanding various oils for the hospital in the *Rab'-i-Rashídí* at Tabríz, where, according to the report of the physician in charge, Muḥammad ibnu'n-Nílí, who is described as the "Galen of our times," they were urgently needed. The quantity of each oil required (varying from 1 to 300 maunds) and the place from which it is to be obtained are carefully specified. Shíráz is to supply six different kinds; Baṣra, seven; Asia Minor, six; Baghdád, nine; Syria, three; and Ḥilla, three. Most of them are aromatic oils prepared from various fragrant flowers, violets, jessamine, narcissus, roses of different sorts, myrtle, orange-blossoms and the like, but we find also absinth, mastic, camomile, castor oil, and even oil of scorpions. In a post-script the writer urges speed in the fulfilment of these commissions, and orders that, to save delay, a separate messenger is to be sent to each of the six localities indicated.

No. 19 (ff. 36 *b*–40 *a*), addressed by Rashíd to his son Amír 'Alí, governor of Baghdád, instructing him as to pensions and presents to be given to learned men throughout the Persian Empire from the Oxus to the Jamna and as far west as Asia Minor and the Egyptian frontiers. The presents in each case consist of a sum of money, a fur cloak or pelisse, and a beast for riding. Only one of the 49 persons named is specifically described as a physician, namely one Maḥmúd ibn Ilyás[1], who is to receive 1000 *dínárs* in cash, a cloak of grey squirrel, and a horse or mule with saddle.

No. 21 (ff. 45 *b*–53 *b*), addressed by Rashíd to his son Jalálu'd-Dín, governor of Asia Minor, requesting him to send every year to Tabríz for use in the hospital quantities varying from 50 to 100 maunds of six drugs, namely, anise-seed, agaric, mastic, lavender, dodder and wormwood.

No. 29 (ff. 87 *b*–92 *a*). This letter was written from Multán in Sind to Mawláná Quṭbu'd-Dín of Shíráz. The writer complains that he had been compelled to abandon his pleasant life in Persia and undertake a troublesome journey to India at the whim of Arghún the Mongol, who wished him to impress on the Indian kings and princes the power and greatness of his master, and at the same time to collect certain useful drugs not to be found in Persia. He expresses satisfaction at the success of his mission and his approaching return home

[1] See **No. 41** *infra.*

and incidentally describes how he succeeded without offending Sulṭán 'Alá'u'd-Dín, to whom he was accredited, in remonstrating with him on his excessive indulgence in wine, the remonstrance being rendered so palatable by an entertaining anecdote and some appropriate verses that his royal host, instead of being annoyed, assigned to him and his son after him a handsome pension.

No. 36 (ff. 120 *b*–131 *b*) is a very long letter, written when Rashíd was suffering from what he believed to be a mortal illness, containing elaborate instructions about the disposal of his property and the maintenance of his foundations. He gives some particulars of the library which he had bequeathed to the *Rab'-i-Rashídí*, comprising 1000 *Qur'áns*, many of them written by the most famous calligraphists, and 60,000 other manuscripts, scientific and literary, including books brought from India and China. He also makes special mention of 1000 Chinese syrup-jars, very artistically made, each bearing the name of the syrup for which it was intended, and Chinese boxes for electuaries.

No. 40 (ff. 136 *a*–138 *b*), though not concerned with medicine, is interesting as showing the solidarity of the Muslim world, the rapidity with which ideas permeated it, even to the remotest parts, and the immense stimulus to learning which one generous patron could give, even in lands not politically connected with his own. It contains Rashíd's instructions to one of his agents in Asia Minor as to the adequate remuneration in money and presents of the learned men in the Maghrib, or western lands of Islám, who had written books in his honour. Of these ten, six were resident in Cordova, Seville and other parts of Andalusia, and four in Tunis, Tripoli and Qayruwán. We flatter ourselves on the facilities of communication existing in these our days, but it is questionable whether an idea, a book, or a philosophical doctrine would travel so quickly now from Tunis to Tabríz or from Seville to Samarqand as it did in the fourteenth century. So potent was the unifying effect of Islám and its universal medium the Arabic language!

No. 41 (ff. 138 *b*–140 *b*) concerns the reconstruction and re-endowment of a hospital at Shíráz, which, originally founded by the Atábeks of Fárs a century earlier, had for some time fallen into decay. Rashíd now appoints a new physician, Mahmúd ibn Ilyás[1], who had attracted his favourable notice by a medical work entitled *Latá'if-i-Rashídiyya* composed in his honour. I do not know whether this book is still extant, but Fonahn[2] mentions another, entitled *Tuhfatu'l-Hukamá* (the "Physicians' Gift"), by the same author, of which there is a manuscript in the *Núr-i-'Uthmániyya* Library at Constantinople. To this physician are hereby assigned a yearly salary and handsome gifts payable from the local revenues, and he is placed in control of the hospital and all its endowments.

No. 42 (ff. 141 *a*–142 *b*) is entirely concerned with the hospital at Hamadán (Rashíd's native city), which had also fallen into an unsatisfactory state through misappropriation of its revenues. A new physician, Ibn Mahdí, is appointed to take charge of the hospital and reorganize it with more regard to the welfare of the patients and the supply of the necessary drugs and medicaments, amongst which special mention is made of several not easily procured, such as Terra sigillata (*tín-i-makhtúm*), Oil of balsam (*rawghan-i-balsán*),

---

[1] See **No. 19** *supra*.

[2] *Zur Quellenkunde d. Pers. Medizin*, p. 124.

Folia Indica or Malabathrum (*sádhaj-i-hindí*), and Theban electuary (*tiryáq-i-fárúq*). Arrangements are also proposed for the proper ordering of the accounts, and the physician, after attending to all these matters, and appointing a dispenser, a dresser, a cook and other officers, is instructed to return to Tabríz, where further favours await him. This letter is one of the few which is dated: it was written from Caesarea (*Qaysariyya*) in A.H. 690 (A.D. 1291).

No. 47 (ff. 151*a*–156*b*) is a letter written from India by Malik 'Alá'u'd-Dín to Rashíd, complimenting him on his public spirit and services to humanity, and containing a long list of presents forwarded to him by the port of Basra. These presents are arranged in twelve categories, viz. (1) wearing apparel, (2) precious stones, (3) perfumes, (4) rare animals, (5) conserves, (6) drugs and simples, (7) a lotion for removing freckles, placed in a class by itself, (8) upholstery, (9) aromatic oils, (10) plate and china, (11) spices and dried fruits, and (12) rare woods and ivory. The list of drugs is the longest and contains 22 items, including cinnamon, nutmeg, cloves, cardamoms, cubebs, cassia, fumitory and betel-nuts.

No. 51 (ff. 171*b*–175*b*). From Rashíd to his son Sa'du'd-Dín, governor of Qinnasrín and the 'Awásim in Asia Minor, describing the concourse of scholars attracted to Tabríz by his bounty and the splendours of the suburb of *Rab'-i-Rashídí*, on which he has lavished so much care and money. It contained 24 caravanserais, 1500 workshops, and 30,000 beautiful houses, besides gardens, baths, shops, mills, weaving and dyeing establishments, paper factories, and a mint. The inhabitants had been carefully chosen from various cities and countries. There were 200 professional *Qur'án-*

readers with fixed salaries to read the scripture daily in the chapel appointed for that purpose and to train forty selected acolytes. There was a Scholars' Street (*Kúcha-i-'ulamá*), where dwelt 400 divines, jurisconsults and traditionists, with suitable salaries and allowances, and in the neighbouring students' quarters lived 1000 eager students from various Muslim countries whose studies were subsidized and directed according to their aptitudes. Fifty skilful physicians had been attracted thither from India, China, Egypt, Syria and other countries, to each of whom were assigned ten enthusiastic students with definite duties in the hospital, to which were also attached surgeons, oculists and bone-setters, each of whom had the charge of five students. All these dwelt in the Street of the Healers (*Kúcha-i-mu'áliján*) at the back of the hospital, near the gardens and orchards of Rashídábád.

I have now completed what I have to say about the history and literature of the so-called Arabian Medicine within the restricted limits imposed on me by considerations of space and time, and I propose now to say a few words about the system itself, with special reference to the *Kámilu's-Siná'at*, or " Liber Regius," of al-Majúsí, the *Qánún* of Avicenna, and especially the Persian " Thesaurus " of Khwárazmsháh, which is accessible only in manuscript. All these three are systematic treatises dealing with the whole science and art of Medicine as understood by the medieval Muslim world. The " Liber Regius " is the simplest in its arrangement, consisting of two volumes each containing ten Discourses (*Maqála*), the first ten dealing with the theory and the second ten with the practice of Medicine; and its Latin translation, printed at Lyons in 1523, is the best and most adequate of these translations which

I have met with. The other two books suffer from the common Oriental fault of exaggerated and over-elaborate subdivision. Ignoring these, the contents of the ten books (*i.e.* nine books and a supplement) which constitute the "Thesaurus" are briefly as follows:

Book I, comprising 6 Discourses and 77 chapters, treats of the definition, scope and utility of Medicine; of the Natures, Elements, Complexions or Temperaments and Humours; of Anatomy, general and special; and of the three-fold Functions or Powers of the body, natural, animal and psychical.

Book II, comprising 9 Discourses and 151 chapters, treats of health and disease (including General Pathology, classification and nomenclature); signs and symptoms, especially the pulse and the excretions; aetiology; Embryology and Obstetric Medicine and the growth and care of the child; the emotions; and Life and Death.

Book III, comprising 14 Discourses and 204 chapters, treats of Hygiene, including the effects of climate, season, air, water, food and drink of all kinds, especially wine; sleeping, waking, movement and rest; clothing and perfumes; bleeding, purging and emetics; dyscrasia; mental states and their effects on the body; the prodromata of disease; and the care of children, the aged and travellers.

Book IV, comprising 4 Discourses and 25 chapters, treats of the importance and principles of diagnosis, and of coction, crisis and prognosis.

Book V, comprising 6 Discourses and 80 chapters, treats of the varieties, aetiology, symptoms and treatment of Fever, the first four Discourses being chiefly devoted to malarial fevers, the fifth to small-pox and measles, and the sixth to recurrence, prophylaxis, diet, and the treatment of convalescents.

Book VI, comprising 21 Discourses and 434 chapters, treats of local diseases *a capite ad calcem*, including mental affections, epilepsy, apoplexy, paralysis, tetanus, dropsy, gynaecology, obstetrics, gout, rheumatism, sciatica and elephantiasis.

Book VII, comprising 7 Discourses and 55 chapters, treats of general pathological conditions which may affect any organ, including tumours, abscesses, cancer, wounds, fractures and dislocations, and contains a Discourse of 12 chapters on the use of the actual cautery.

Book VIII, comprising 3 Discourses and 37 chapters, treats of personal cleanliness and the care of the hair, nails and complexion.

Book IX, comprising 5 Discourses and 44 chapters, treats of poisons, animal, vegetable, and mineral; and of the bites and stings of beasts, snakes and venomous reptiles and insects.

Here this immense work, comprising 9 Books, 75 Discourses, and 1107 chapters, originally ended with the colophon : "*Here endeth the Book of Poisons, with the conclusion of which endeth the Work entitled the Thesaurus of Khwárazmsháh, by the Favour of God and His Help,*" but there follow three final sections of apology, the first for delay in completing the book, the second for its defects, and the third for all physicians who themselves fall victims to the diseases they treat[1].

Subsequently the author added a Conclusion, or tenth Book, on Materia Medica, divided into three parts, the first dealing with animal products, the second with simple vegetable drugs, and the third with compound medicaments.

---

[1] *Cf.* the Arabic verses on pp. 8 and 9 *supra*, and the foot-note on p. 59.

At this point we may pause to consider two questions which have been constantly present in my mind during the preparation of these lectures. The first question is, how far can the fuller study of Arabian Medicine be regarded as likely to repay the labour it involves? The second question is, supposing it to be worth fuller study, how should that study be pursued in the future, and what parts of the subject most merit attention?

From the narrowest utilitarian point of view it is not likely that even the profoundest study of the subject will yield any practical results of importance, seeing that the whole system is based on a rudimentary Anatomy, an obsolete Physiology, and a fantastic Pathology. From the Arabian Materia Medica and from the rules of Diet and Hygiene some hints might possibly be gleaned; but with this exception we must, I fear, admit that little practical advantage can be hoped for. Few educated people, however, and certainly no one in the distinguished audience I have the honour of addressing, will take this narrow, purely utilitarian view, of which, indeed, the very existence of the Fitz-Patrick Lectures is a negation. That the Embryology of Science, the evolution of our present *Weltanschauung*, is a proper and even a noble subject of research we shall all readily admit; but still the question remains whether the Arabs did more than transmit the wisdom of the Greeks, and whether they added much original matter to the scientific concepts of which for some eight centuries they were the chief custodians. This, unfortunately, is not an easy question to answer, and much laborious research will be needed ere it can be answered definitely. For such research, moreover, a combination of qualifications not very commonly met with in one individual is required, to wit, a scholarly knowledge of Greek, Latin, Syriac, Arabic and Persian, and, if possible, Sanskrit; a knowledge of, or at least an interest in Medicine; abundant leisure; voracious and omnivorous reading; and great enthusiasm and industry. And it must be said once and for all that no just idea of Arabian Medicine can be derived from the very imperfect Latin renderings of the standard Arabic works. I gave one example in a previous lecture of the unintelligible transcription of Arabic words, evidently not understood, into Latin, and I will now give another. In the Latin translation of the *Qánún* of Avicenna printed at Venice in 1544, on f. 198 *a* you will find, under diseases of the head and brain, a section entitled "*Sermo universalis de Karabito qui est apostema capitis sirsem.*" If you refer to the corresponding passage of the Arabic text (p. 302) printed at Rome in 1593, you will find this mysterious disease appearing as *qaránítus* (قرانيطس). But the true reading, given in a fine old MS. which I recently acquired, is *farránítis* (فرانيطس), that is φρενῖτις, frensy. Such is the havoc wrought in Arabic letters by the misplacement of dots and diacritical points, and in the case of these unfamiliar Greek words there is nothing to guide the Arabian scribe if the word be indistinctly written, one form appearing as intelligible or as unintelligible as another. Hence the student of Arabic medical literature must begin by correcting and re-editing even the printed texts before he can begin to read or translate them; and the numerous important books which exist only in manuscript will, of course, give him still more trouble, since to consult what still survives of the *Ḥáwí* or "Continens" of Rází—the most important as well as the most voluminous Arabic work on Medicine—he will have to visit not only the

British Museum and the Bodleian Libraries, but Munich and the Escorial, and even then he will not have seen half of this great work. Nor is there much hope that critical editions of these books will ever be published unless Egyptian medical students or young Indian scholars with a taste for research and a desire to render service to the renown of Islamic science can be stimulated by material and moral support to undertake this laborious and un-remunerative but important work. As an example of what may be done by such workers, I desire to call attention to Mawlawí 'Azímu'd-Dín 'Ahmad's admirable *Catalogue of the Arabic Medical Works in the Oriental Public Library at Bankipore* (Calcutta, 1910), a fine and scholarly piece of work carried out at the instigation and under the supervision of Sir E. Denison Ross, at that time Director of the Muhammadan Madrasa at Calcutta, but now of the London School of Oriental Studies.

Apart from new elements, not of Greek origin, which may be disclosed by a more minute and atten-tive study of Arabian Medicine, there is the practical certainty that the seven books of Galen's *Anatomy*, lost in the original, but preserved in an Arabic trans-lation and published with a German translation by Dr Max Simon in 1906, are not the only ancient medical works of which the substance if not the form may be recovered in this way. And we must further remember that the Arab translators, who were at work nearly 1200 years ago, were in contact with a living tradition which went back from Baghdád to Jundí-Shápúr, thence to Edessa and Antioch, and thence to Alexandria; and that this tradition may well serve to elucidate many obscure points in the Greek texts still preserved to us. Finally the clinical observations (embodied especially in the works of Rází) have an intrinsic value of their own which would undoubtedly repay investigation. On all these grounds, then, even if we rate the originality of Arabian Medicine at the lowest, I venture to think that it well deserves more careful and systematic study.

In considering medieval science as a whole we cannot fail to be struck by two peculiarities which it presents, the solidarity and interdependence of all its branches, and the dominance of certain numbers in its basic conceptions. The sum of knowledge was not then so immense as to defy comprehension by one individual, and it is seldom that we find a medieval physician content to confine his attention exclusively to the medical sciences, or unwilling to include in his studies astronomy and astrology, music and mathematics, and even ethics, metaphysics and politics. It is said in the *Qur'án* (xli, 53): "*We will show them Our signs in the horizon and in themselves,*" and this has encouraged many of the mystically-minded amongst the Muslims to seek for correspondences not only between stars, plants, bodies and the like, but between the material and spiritual worlds. The strange sect of the Isma'ílís or Esoterics (*Bátiniyya*), out of which were developed the notorious Assassins, instructed their missionaries to arouse the curiosity of the potential proselyte by such questions as "Why has a man seven cervical and twelve dorsal vertebrae?" "Why has each of the fingers three joints, but the thumb only two?" and the like; and it was to them a fact of infinite significance that the number of joints on the two hands agreed with the number of permanent teeth, the number of days in the lunar month, and the number of letters in the Arabic alphabet. So in their cosmogony we notice the great part played by the numbers four, seven and twelve. Thus we have the four Natural Properties, Heat, Cold, Dryness and Moisture; the four Elements; the four Seasons; the four Humours; the four Winds, and the like. Also the seven Planets, the seven Climes, the seven Days of the Week, and the seven Seas; the twelve Signs of the Zodiac, the twelve Months of the Year, and so on.

According to the conception of the oldest Arabian physicians, it is the four Natural Properties rather than what are commonly called the four Elements which are really elemental. This is very plainly stated by 'Alí ibn Rabban aṭ-Ṭabarí in the third chapter of his "Paradise of Wisdom," where he says:

" The simple Natures called elemental are four, two active, to wit, Heat and Cold, and two passive, to wit, Moisture and Dryness. And the Compound Natures also are four, and the fact that they are called ' compound ' shows that the simple ones precede them, since the compound originates from the simple. Of these Compound Natures the first is Fire, which is hot, dry, light, and centrifugal in movement; the second Air, which is hot, moist and light, moving or blowing in every direction; the third Water, which is cold, moist, heavy, and centripetal in movement; and the fourth Earth, which is cold, dry and heavy, and moves ever towards the lowest.... All earthly substances are subordinate to the Fire, and are affected and changed by it. And the Natural Properties are four, because the Agent becomes active only through the Object on which it acts. The two active Natural Principles are Heat and Cold, whereof each has its own proper object, whence the Four."

" These Natures," continues our author in the next chapter, "are mutually hostile and antagonistic, and most violently so when this antagonism arises simultaneously from two sides or aspects; as, for instance, in the case of Fire, which is antagonistic both by its Heat and Dryness to the Cold and Moisture of Water; or Air, which is antagonistic both by its Heat and Moisture to the Cold and Dryness of Earth. But if the antagonism be on one side only, it is less pronounced, as, for instance, in the case of Air, which is opposed to Water by its Heat, but agrees with it in its Moisture. Therefore hath God made the Air a barrier between the Water and the Fire, and the Water a barrier between the Earth and the Air."

Here follows a diagram which may be further amplified from the *Kitábu't-tanbíh* ("Livre d'Avertissement")[1] of the great historian and geographer Mas'údí, who wrote in the middle of the tenth century of our era. In this diagram Heat opposed to Cold and Dryness opposed to Moisture constitute the four cardinal points. Compounded of Heat and Dryness on the different Planes or orders of Phenomena are Fire of the Four Elements, Summer of the Four Seasons, the South of the Four Regions, Youth of the Four Ages of Man, and the Yellow Bile of the Four Humours. Similarly from Dryness and Cold we have Earth, Autumn, the West, the Mature Age, and the Black Bile; from Cold and Moisture, Water, Winter, the North, Old Age and the Phlegm; and from Heat and Moisture, Air, Spring, the East, Childhood and the Blood.

The Universe or Macrocosm, according to this conception, comprises the Earth or Terrestrial Sphere

---

[1] The Arabic text, printed at Leyden in 1894, constitutes vol. viii of the late Professor de Goeje's *Bibliotheca Geographorum Arabicorum.* The French translation by Carra de Vaux was published in Paris in 1896 under the title *Le Livre de l'Avertissement et de la Revision.*

surrounded by twelve concentric enveloping spheres,
namely, the Aqueous, Aerial and Igneous Spheres, the
Seven Planetary Spheres, beginning with that of the
Moon and ending with that of Saturn, the Zodiacal
Sphere or Sphere of the Fixed Stars, and outside all
the *Falaku'l-Aflák* ("the Heaven of the Heavens") or
al-Falaku'l-Aṭlas ("the Plain," or Starless, "Heaven"),
the Empyrean of Ptolemy, beyond which, according to
the common opinion, is *al-Khalá,* "the Vacuum," or *Lá
Khalá wa lá Malá,* "neither Vacuum nor Plenum." The
generation of terrestrial existences is supposed to have
been brought about by the interaction of the Seven
Planets, or "Seven Celestial Sires," and the Four
Elements, or "Four Terrestrial Mothers," from which
resulted the "Threefold Progeny," or the Mineral, Vegetable and Animal Kingdoms. The first of these was
produced in the interspace between the Terrestrial and
the Aqueous Spheres, the second between the Aqueous
and Aerial Spheres, and the third between the Aerial
and Igneous Spheres. The process of Evolution from
Mineral to Plant, from Plant to Animal and from Animal
to Man is clearly recognized, and is fully discussed by
Dieterici in the ninth book of his exposition of Arabian
Philosophy, as taught by the encyclopaedists of Baghdád
in the ninth and tenth centuries of our era, entitled
*Der Darwinismus im zehnten und neunzehnten Jahr-
hundert*[1]. In the twelfth-century Persian work entitled
the "Four Discourses," which I have already had
occasion to cite, attempts are even made to identify the
"missing links," coral being regarded as intermediate
between the mineral and vegetable kingdoms; the vine,
which seeks to avoid and escape from the fatal embrace
of a kind of bind-weed called *'ashaqa,* as intermediate

[1] Leipzig, 1878.

between the vegetable and animal kingdoms; and the *nasnás*, a kind of ape or wild man, as intermediate between man and the beasts.

The general principles which constitute the basis of Arabian Medicine are the outcome of these conceptions, and the opening chapters of every great systematic work on the subject deal largely with the doctrine of the "Temperaments" or "Complexions" (*Mizáj*, plural *Amzija*), the Natural Properties (*Tabáyi'*), and the Humours (*Akhlát*). *Mizáj*, which is still the common word for health in Arabic, Persian and Turkish, is derived from a root meaning "to mix," and indicates a state of equilibrium between the four Natural Properties or the four Humours; while if this equilibrium is upset by the preponderance of one of the Natural Properties or the Humours, a disturbance entitled *Inhiráfu'l-Mizáj*, or "Deflection of the temperamental equilibrium," is produced. But even the normal healthy *Mizáj* is not practically a constant quantity, each region, season, age, individual and organ having its own special and appropriate type. Nine types of Complexion are recognized, namely the equable (*mu'tadil*), which is practically non-existent; the four simple Complexions, hot, cold, dry and moist; and the four compound, namely the hot and dry, the hot and moist, the cold and dry, and the cold and moist. Excluding the rare case of a perfect equilibrium, every individual will be either of the Bilious Complexion, which is hot and dry; the Atrabilious or Melancholic, which is cold and dry; the Phlegmatic, which is cold and moist; or the Sanguine, which is hot and moist. In treating a hot, cold, dry or moist disease with a food or drug of the opposite quality, regard must be paid to these idiosyncrasies. The Natural Property inherent in each food or drug exists in one of four degrees. Thus, for example, such a substance if hot in the first degree is a food; if hot in the second degree, both a food and a medicine; if hot in the third degree, a medicine, not a food; if hot in the fourth degree, a poison. Another four-fold division of substances which react on the human body is into those which act beneficially both internally and externally, like wheat, which in the stomach is a food and externally a poultice to "ripen" wounds or sores; those which are beneficial internally but mischievous externally, like garlic, which, taken internally, increases the natural Heat, but applied externally acts as a poison; those which are poisons internally but antidotes externally, like Litharge (*Murdásang*) and Verdigris or Acetate of Copper (*Zangár*); and lastly those which both externally and internally act as poisons, like Aconite (*Bísh*) and Ergot (*Qurún-i-Sunbul*).

The third Discourse (*Guftár*) of the First Book of the "Thesaurus" is devoted to the discussion of the four Humours. It comprises six chapters, four treating in turn of each of the Humours, one (the first) of their nature, and one (the last) of their production and differentiation. The first chapter is so short that it may be translated in full. "Humour," says the author, "is a moisture circulating in the human body and naturally located in the veins and hollow organs, such as the stomach, liver, spleen and gall-bladder; and it is produced from the food. Some Humours are good and some bad. The good are those which nourish man's body and take the place of the fluids which are expended. The bad are those which are useless for this purpose, and these are the Humours of which the body must be cleansed by drugs. The Humours are four, Blood, Phlegm, Yellow Bile and Black Bile." According to al-Majúsí's "Liber Regius" they are the proximate, or secondary, and special elements (*ustuqussát,* στοιχεῖα) of the bodies of all warm-blooded animals, as contrasted with the remote, or primary, and common elements, Earth, Air, Fire and Water, with which they severally correspond, as already explained, and from which they arise, being therefore called the "Daughters of the Elements" (*Banátu'l-Arkán*).

Stated briefly, the theory of the production and distribution of the four Humours is as follows. In the stomach the food undergoes a "first digestion" whereby the more nutritious part of it is converted into chyle, called by the Arabs *Kaylús*; but, besides the unnutritious residue which is rejected, a portion is converted into Phlegm, which differs from the other three Humours in having no special location, such as the Blood has in the liver, the Yellow Bile in the gall-bladder, and the Black Bile in the spleen. The chyle is conveyed to the liver by the portal vein, which receives the veins of the stomach and mesentery, and there it undergoes a "second digestion" or coction, which divides it into three portions, a scum or froth which is the Yellow Bile; a sediment, which is the Black Bile; and the Blood, which contains its choicest ingredients. The Blood passes on by the Superior Vena Cava to the heart, having dismissed its more aqueous part to the kidneys for excretion, and is thence distributed by the arteries to the various organs, in which it undergoes a fourth and final coction or "digestion" (the third having taken place in the blood-vessels). In the normal body the Humours exist in a state of mixture, save that a reserve of Yellow Bile is stored in the gall-bladder and of Black Bile in the spleen; but the separation and elimination of any Humour can be effected by appropriate therapeutic agents, drugs or otherwise. Each Humour may be natural and normal, or unnatural and abnormal. The normal Blood is of two kinds, the one dark red and thick, occurring in the liver and veins; the other moister, warmer, more fluid, and of a brighter red, occurring in the heart and arteries. Blood may become abnormal simply through excess of heat or cold, or by admixture with superfluous bilious, atrabilious or phlegmatic matter. Of the Phlegm four abnormal qualities are recognized, the aqueous, the mucous, the vitreous and the calcareous; and of the Yellow Bile the same number.

Here follow, alike in the *Qánún* and the "Thesaurus," the sections dealing with general and special Anatomy, the subject-matter of which is accessible to the general reader in Dr P. de Koning's excellent work *Trois traités d'Anatomie Arabes.* Thanks to him and to Dr Max Simon, this branch of Arabian Medicine has been more thoroughly elucidated than any other, and I may therefore pass on to the sections on the Natural Functions and Virtues, or Faculties, which complete what may be called the General Physiology of the Arabian physicians. These Functions or Virtues are primarily divided into three classes, the Natural, common to the Animal and Vegetable kingdoms; the Animal, peculiar to the Animal kingdom; and the Psychical, some of which are common to man and the higher animals, while others are peculiar to man. The Natural Virtues are the Nutritive and the Reproductive, the first including the Attractive, Retentive, Digestive and Expulsive. The Animal Virtues or Functions are the active, connected with the phenomena of Respiration and Circulation, and the passive, connected with the simpler emotions of Fear, Anger, Disgust, and the like, common to men and animals. The Psychic Virtues or Functions include motor or sensory powers common to all animals, and the higher mental faculties, Thought, Memory, Imagination and the like, peculiar to man. Corresponding with the Five External Senses, Taste, Touch, Hearing, Smelling and Seeing, are the Five Internal Senses, of which the first and second, the compound sense (or "Sensus Communis") and the Imagination, are located in the anterior ventricle of the brain; the third and fourth, the Co-ordinating and Emotional Faculties, in the mid-brain; and the fifth, the Memory, in the hind-brain[1]. Here there exists some confusion between the nomenclature adopted by physicians and metaphysicians, which Avicenna especially emphasizes, impressing on the former, to whom his *Qánún* is addressed, that their concern is less with abstract philosophical ideas than with what lies within the scope of actual practice.

Here I should like to call your attention to a rather remarkable passage[2] in the *Kitábu'l-Malikí*, or "Liber Regius," of 'Alí ibnu'l-'Abbás al-Majúsí, who died in A.D. 982, about the time when Avicenna was born. This passage, which occurs in the chapter treating of the Animal Virtues or Vital Functions, deals chiefly with the two opposite movements of expansion (*inbisát*) and contraction (*inqibád*), which in the heart and arteries constitute diastole and systole, and in the respiratory organs inspiration and expiration. These movements are compared to those of a bellows, except that they are produced by an internal, not by an external, force; and it is, of course, supposed by the writer that the heart draws air from the lungs to mix with the blood for the elaboration of the Vital Spirit, just as the lungs inhale it from without, and that the "vaporized superfluities" (*al-fudúlu'd-dukhániyya*), or vitiated air, are expelled by

[1] See my *Year amongst the Persians*, pp. 144–5.
[2] Vol. i, pp. 138–9 of the Cairo edition.

the reverse process. Having concluded his remarks on Respiration, the author continues as follows:

" And you must know that during the diastole such of the pulsating vessels (*i.e.* the arteries) as are near the heart draw in air and sublimated blood from the heart by compulsion of vacuum, because during the systole they are emptied of blood and air, but during the diastole the blood and air return and fill them. Such of them as are near the skin draw air from the outer atmosphere; while such as are intermediate in position between the heart and the skin have the property of drawing from the non-pulsating vessels (*i.e.* the veins) the finest and most subtle of the blood. This is because in the non-pulsating vessels (*i.e.* the veins) are pores communicating with the pulsating vessels (*i.e.* the arteries). The proof of this is that when an artery is cut, all the blood which is in the veins also is evacuated."

Here, as it seems to me, we clearly have a rudimentary conception of the capillary system.

Corresponding with the three categories of Faculties or Virtues are three Spirits, the Natural, the Animal and the Psychical, the first elaborated in the Liver and thence conveyed by the Veins to the Heart; the second elaborated in the Heart and conveyed by the carotid arteries to the Brain, and the third elaborated in the Brain and thence conveyed by the nerves to all parts of the body. These, and their relation one to another, and to the immortal Spirit or Intelligence of which the existence is generally recognized, are but briefly discussed by Avicenna and the other medical writers whom I have chiefly cited. The fullest discussion of these matters, appertaining rather to Philosophy and Psychology than Medicine, I have found in a very rare Arabic work on the generation and development of man by Abu'l-Ḥasan Saʿíd ibn Hibatu'lláh, court-physician to the Caliph al-Muqtaḍí, who flourished in the second half of the eleventh century[1]. This work entitled *Maqála fí Khalqi'l-Insán* ("Discourse on the Creation of Man") deals chiefly with the processes of Reproduction, Gestation, Parturition, Growth and Decay, but the last ten of the fifty chapters into which it is divided deal with Psychology, including arguments in favour of the survival of Intelligence after Death and against Metempsychosis. The life of the body, according to this writer, depends on the Animal Spirit and ends with its departure "through the channels whereby the air reaches the Heart," *i.e.* through the mouth and nostrils. This conception is embodied in the common Arabic phrase *Mát^a ḥatf^a anfi-hi*, "He died a nose-death," *i.e.* a natural death, the Animal Spirit escaping through the nose and not through a wound. So also we have the common Persian expression *Ján bar lab ámada*, meaning one whose spirit has reached his lips and is on the brink of departure.

My allotted hour runs out, and I must conclude this very inadequate sketch of Arabian Medicine which it has been my privilege and my pleasure to present to you. I hope that you may have found in it, if not much useful instruction, at least a little entertainment. With great misgiving and some unwillingness I undertook the task at the instigation of my teacher and friend Sir Norman Moore, the President of this College, to whose inspiration I owe so much since my student days in St Bartholomew's Hospital. I have been amply rewarded by the task itself, and it shall not be my fault if it is

---

[1] His life is given by Ibn Abí Uṣaybiʿa in his *Classes of Physicians* (vol. i, pp. 254–5 of the Cairo edition).

laid aside because its immediate purpose is fulfilled. More remains to be accomplished in this branch of Arabic studies than in any other of equal importance and much pioneer work is required ere we can hope to reach the ultimate conclusions which are so important for the history of scientific thought throughout the ages. Above all there has grown in me while communing with the minds of these old Arabian and Persian physicians a realization of the solidarity of the human intelligence beyond all limitations of race, space or time, and of the essential nobility of the great profession represented by this College.

INDEX

A hyphen prefixed to a name or word indicates that it should be preceded by the Arabic definite article al-. The prefixes Abú ("father of..."), Ibn ("son of..."), Umm ("mother of...") in Arabic, and de, le, von in European names, are disregarded in the alphabetical arrangement. Names common to two or more persons mentioned in the text are, to save repetition, grouped under one heading, which, in these cases, is printed in Clarendon type, as are the more important reference numbers. Arabic and Persian words and titles of books are printed in *italics*. Roman numbers following a name indicate the century of the Christian era in which the person flourished or the book was written.